FRONTIERS OF PRIMARY CARE

Series Editor: Mack Lipkin, Jr.

D1194346

Frontiers of Primary Care

Series Editor: Mack Lipkin, Jr.

Published Volumes

Barnes, Aronson, and Delbanco (eds.)
  Alcoholism: A Guide for the Primary Care Physician
Schmidt, Lipkin, Jr., de Vries, and Greep (eds.)
  *New Directions for Medical Education: Problem-Based Learning and
  Community-Oriented Medical Education*
Goldbloom and Lawrence (eds.)
  Preventing Disease: Beyond the Rhetoric
WONCA Classification Committee
  Functional Status Measurement in Primary Care

Forthcoming Volumes

Lipkin, Jr., Putnam, and Lazare (eds.)
  The Medical Interview

WONCA Classification Committee

Functional Status Measurement in Primary Care

Foreword by Sheldon Greenfield

With Contributions by M. Baker, J. Barrand, B.G. Bentsen, N. Bentzen, W.J.H.M. van den Bosch, C. Bridges-Webb, T. Christiansen, R.T. Connis, J. Craenen, M-B. De Munter, L. Dessers, R.W. Elford, J. Froom, M.J. Gordon, K. Haepers, R.D. Hays, J. Heyrman, A. Keller, J.W. Kirk, H. Lamberts, J.M. Landgraf, J.E. Liljenquist, R.S. Mecklenberg, B. Meyboom-de Jong, M.H. Mirza, E.C. Nelson, K.M. Pedersen, T.B. Rogers, H. Shigemoto, R.J.A. Smith, A.J.A. Smits, J.W. Stephens, A.L. Stewart, T.R. Taylor, C. van Weel, J.H. Wasson, S.R. West, R.C. Westbury, M. Zubkoff

Springer-Verlag
New York Berlin Heidelberg
London Paris Tokyo Hong Kong

Series Editor
Mack Lipkin, Jr., M.D.
Director, Primary Care;
Associate Professor of Medicine,
New York University Medical Center,
  School of Medicine,
New York, NY 10016, USA

RA407
A2
F86
1990

With 63 Figures

Library of Congress Cataloging-in-Publication Data
Functional status measurement in primary care: report of the
  Classification Committee of WONCA (World Organization of National
  Colleges, Academies, and Academic Associations of General
  Practice/Family Physicians)
      p. cm.--(Frontiers of primary care)
  Papers delivered at a meeting in Calgary Canada, Oct. 24–28, 1988,
  sponsored by WONCA, College of Family Physicians of Canada, and the
  Dept. of Family Medicine, University of Calgary.
    Includes bibliographical references.
    ISBN 0-387-97198-X
    1. Health status indicators--Congresses.   I. World Organization of National Colleges,
  Academies, and Academic Associations of General Practitioners/Family
  Physicians Classification Committee. II. College of Family
  Physicians of Canada. III. University of Calgary. Dept. of Family
  Medicine. IV. Series.
    [DNLM: 1. Activities of Daily Living--congresses. 2. Health
  Surveys--congresses. 3. Primary Health Care--congresses. W 84.6
  F979 1988]
  RA407.A2F86 1990
  362.1--dc20
  DNLM/DLC
  for Library of Congress   89-26345

Printed on acid-free paper.

Typeset by Thomson Press (India) Limited, New Delhi, India.
Printed and bound by Edwards Brothers, Inc., Ann Arbor, Michigan,
Printed in the United States of America.

9 8 7 6 5 4 3 2 1

ISBN 0-387-97198-X Springer-Verlag New York Berlin Heidelberg
ISBN 3-540-97198-X Springer-Verlag Berlin Heidelberg New York

These papers were delivered at a meeting in Calgary, Canada October 24–28, 1988. Meeting sponsored by the World Organization of National Colleges, Academies, and Academic Associations of General Practice/Family Physicians (WONCA); The College of Family Physicians of Canada; and The Department of Family Medicine of the University of Calgary, Canada.

The Classification Committee of WONCA gratefully acknowledges financial assistance for this workshop from The Alberta Heritage Foundation for Medical Research, Smith Kline and French Canada, Ltd., and The Department of Family Medicine of the University of Calgary, Canada.

Series Preface

Primary care medicine is a new frontier of medicine. Physicians and scholars in primary care are pioneering new ways to improve health, lessen illness, and make care available and affordable for all. Every nation in the world has recognized the necessity to deliver personal and primary care to its people. Primary care has come to mean first contact care based on a positive caring relationship between an individual patient and a single provider who manages the majority of a patient's problems, coordination and advocacy for all the patient's care, and the provision of preventive and psychosocial care as well as care for episodes of acute and chronic illness. These facets of care work most effectively when they are embedded in a coherent, integrated approach.

The impetus for support of primary care derived from several trends. First, the costs of care based in new technologies rocketed beyond ability to pay and no clear rational approach to prioritization of expenditures emerged. This was exacerbated by expanding populations and diminished real resources in many regions.

Simultaneously, the primary care disciplines have grown into mature disciplines with new intellectual and clinical tools to offer in place of more costly and often dehumanized approaches. The intellectual tools include clinical epidemiology that examines the efficacy, effectiveness, and efficiency of every day real world care; clinical decision making, which is finding new ways to enhance the rational basis of every day clinical choice; the medical interview, the major medium of care which is now undergoing scientific scrutiny and refinement; problem based learning and community based medical education, which are enabling efficient learning of the greatest relevance for practice and providing heightened satisfaction for both student and teacher; and the philosophic and empiric study of ethical aspects of care.

The emergence of these new disciplines within primary care has prompted a series of ongoing questions. Who is to do primary care and with what preparation? What are the knowledge, skills, and attitudes needed in practitioners and teachers of primary care? What research or teaching and clinical methods are available and what are their strengths and weaknesses?

Frontiers of Primary Care plans to help meet the needs of primary care professionals and their students by reporting about fundamental and applied research findings in clinically relevant, readable ways. It will provide teachers and clinicians with necessary information about such areas as alcoholism, the medical interview, prevention, and functional assessment of the patient.

This volume will serve the needs of both researchers interested in clinical assessment of the function of patients and clinicians who need ways to monitor how their patients are doing with respect to goals of treatment (in addition to the biologic markers of disease). It exemplifies how the community of generalists are working together to develop needed clinical tools. It points to both present applications of the functional assessment approach and to ongoing research needed to further validate and refine these methods.

Mack Lipkin, Jr.
Series Editor

Foreword

This book represents two extraordinary initiatives. First, it brings together the nations of the world to focus on a critical but heretofore uncharted territory: the standardization of measurement of clinical health, as contrasted to public health on one hand and biological science on the other. It is a far from new occurrence to have a group of oncologists get together at an international meeting to decide on a classification scheme for lymphomas. On the other hand, who has fostered statistics and international comparisons with respect to crude public health measures such as infant mortality? This volume heralds a movement to bring together the physicians of the world on a care level, not a biological, public health, or even epidemiological level. The proposed mechanism to fill that gap is called functional status, which WONCA (World Organization of National Colleges, Academies, and Academic Associations of General Practioners/Family Physicians) has put forward as a standardizable universal that physicians and patients can recognize as part of what they do every day. Standardization through these functional status measures, a goal that this book advances, will allow comparisons and transfer of advances in quality of care, medical education, and cost/resources control that will improve care and unite family and other general physicians.

Not only is the choice of functional status good because it represents the goal of family physicians and generalists everywhere, but in addition, this summary measure also potentially reflects the aim of generalists to create the most appropriate and least expensive balance between technical care and interpersonal care. To the degree that functional status measures, which are reported by the patient, represent both technical care and interpersonal care, they document the true role of the generalist in this very complex specialist oriented society. This set of goals is expressed in the WONCA classification, but the inclusion of functional status measurements allows this classification to come alive and to measure and test whether the elements of this classification make sense in daily practice and whether they are being carried out at an optimal level.

The second virtue of this volume and the Calgary conference from which it has evolved is the bringing together of pure researchers in psychometrics and measurement on one hand, with physicians who practice or head up units and use their own practices as testing grounds for reality on the other. The inclusion in this volume of case reports which suggest acceptability for these instruments represents a nice juxtaposition of clinical sensibility with the use of psychometric maneuvers such as factor analysis to develop and test the instruments. The introductory chapters by Stuart and Rogers set a solid groundwork for a field about which most clinicians are naïve and in fact could benefit from with respect to physiologic measures, which do not often meet good measurement standards. Trials in different countries in different units indicate good supporting data for early acceptance of these instruments by family physicians. Perhaps the most extensive trials have been with the Dartmouth Coop Charts, which show some very promising results toward a goal of international classification. Whether or not this goal is achieved through those charts or other health status measures, consideration of universal standards, even with different instruments, opens the way to the standardizations and comparisons and ultimately training that are necessary.

The Health Status Conferences sponsored by the Henry J. Kaiser Family Foundation and the Institute of Medicine called "Advances in Health Status Assessment," have shown remarkable convergence of instruments, despite the fact that the originators of these instruments built them on what initially appeared to be rather disparate, conceptual foundations. Despite some differences, particularly in administration and inclusion or exclusion of various dimensions, this remarkable convergence of instruments, is indicated in this volume.

Is the glass half full or is the glass half empty? Where do we stand and where does this volume tell us we stand with respect to the creation and use of functional status instruments? In many respects we have come quite far as indicated here, but what is left to do? One of the striking needs expressed by members of WONCA and authors in this book is the need for a short easily administered form that can be well integrated into generalists' practices. One of the great virtues of the Dartmouth Coop Charts, as well as other measures, is that they are short. It is important, however, to address the trade-off between short instruments and those Rogers refers to as a "wider band," i.e., longer, more precise instruments. It may be, for example, that the functional status instruments might be better used every six months with a longer version that supplies more generalizeable and more comparative information with shorter forms being used in between. The trade-offs between the short form and longer forms, a topic that Nelson et al. address, needs to be understood better before this issue of the trade-off is fully appreciated.

A second issue surrounding the relationship of these measures to clinical health states is still to be determined. There is much work in this book relating functional status measures to various diagnoses, but for a doctor, what is as critical is the patient's level of severity of disease within a diagnosis. A diabetic patient with high blood sugar and no complications is much more like a normal person or a person with mild hypertension than they are like a severe diabetic with heart, eye, and kidney disease in terms of functional status and total disease burden. Parsing out the amount of patient dysfunction due to disease severity vis-à-vis psychosocial causes will guide the physician's attention to either technical or interpersonal care or to some combination of both. Just as we need to relate blood sugar to hemoglobin A1, BUN to creatinine, chest x-ray for heart size to ejection fraction, symptoms of shortness of breath and dyspnea exertion to heart size, so too do we need to relate functional status measures to clinical measures so that the doctor can understand the patient's combined clinical and functional state.

A third question, suggested in many of these chapters, is how are doctors going to respond to functional status data? Many of the doctors reported that they liked the measures and that they provided new information. However, will that information improve the patient's functional status or the relationship between doctor and patient, or anything that we can measure? Fourth, can we relate these functional status measures to costs of care? If patients achieve similar functional status and some physicians or systems or specialties are spending a lot more money and using a lot more resources, interventions can be designed based upon that information. Fifth, can we make international comparisons or even comparisons within a country of different socioeconomic status groups with measurements that are adjusted for socioeconomic and cultural variables so that we can interpret them more clearly.

These are but some of the future questions that could not even be raised or addressed were it not for the kind of information presented in this book and the level of consensus achieved with respect to the importance and need for functional status information. The continued work of those visionary people who brought about the Calgary Conference and who authored chapters for this book will be critical to our future understanding of the relationship of functional status to resource utilization, to medical education, to the doctor-patient relationship, to cultural differences, and to all the understanding and wisdom that we can gain to improve the quality of medical care.

Sheldon Greenfield

Preface

WONCA Committee on International Classification Statement on Functional Status Assessment, Calgary, October 1988

1. The WONCA Classification Committee will focus on functional status rather than health status or quality of life, although it recognizes that these three concepts are related. The Classification Committee will continue to employ the definition of function, which is "function is the ability of a person to perform and adapt to the individual's given environment, measured both objectively and subjectively over a stated period of time."
2. Functional status measurements must relate directly to current classifications that the committee has produced which include ICHPPC-2-Defined, IC-Process-PC, ICPC, and the International Glossary for Primary Care.
3. Functional status indicators are not identical with objective findings, although objective findings may be used to measure function.
4. Work on functional status assessment is a logical consequence as well as a necessary sequential task which builds on the committee's earlier work to completely define the content of the primary care encounter.
5. A classification of functional status instruments is unlikely to be useful to family physicians. Instead a method of incorporating functional status assessment into clinical practice as well as relating different functional status assessment tools to each other in a hierarchical fashion will be attempted.
6. Several elements must be considered when designing an instrument for use in primary care. These are: assessment of function must be related to the components of the primary care encounter including reason for encounter, diagnosis, process, and others; the time intervals at which functional status is to be assessed must be stated; notation of differences and similarities between assessments by the patient and by the physician is necessary; use of the instruments must be feasible by primary care providers during the routine care of their patients in the ambulatory care setting; the relation-

ship between intervention and a change in function should be understood in clinical terms; instruments employed should be sensitive to the measurement of small changes in function, as well as larger changes expected to occur in more seriously ill patients or rapidly progressing conditions; the use of functional status instruments should facilitate the assessment of outcome; in general several scores derived from the measurement of the several components of function are preferred to aggregate single scores; and validity and reliability assessments of any instruments employed should be as high as possible.

7. Instruments selected should appeal to busy physicians.
8. The committee must keep lines of communication open to social scientists and other disciplines interested in the assessment of patient's function.
9. It is desirable to have some indicators of severity of disease. Functional status may play a role in severity assessment.

The committee considered elements of function which should be measured. These include physical, mental, and social dimensions. Under the physical dimensions are included activities of daily living which are the necessary daily tasks such as bathing, transferring, mobility, eating, dressing, and continence.

The committee considered how the Dartmouth COOP charts fulfilled these several requirements in accord with the principles enunciated above and the needs of the international community. Clearly these charts were attractive to the committee for several reasons. These are: the charts have been demonstrated to have a high level of reliability and validity; they have been demonstrated to have been useful and acceptable in the U.S., The Netherlands, Japan, and Canada; they can be self-administered or administered by a health provider; the time of administration is brief; and the accompanying drawings were felt to aid in understanding (particularly cross-cultural), although the drawings were not attractive to all persons who received the tests.

The physical function assessment is linked to cardiovascular fitness without adjustment for age. Thus this is an absolute rather than a relative measure. The emotional charts describe feeling but fail to measure cognitive function. The daily work chart relates to one's major role or job. The social activities assessment includes social functions outside of one's self but only as related to limitations caused by impaired physical and emotional health. These first four charts therefore are functional measures. Additional charts do not relate to function. The pain chart simply measures pain rather than functional impairment. The change in condition chart was developed to measure the course of illness over time. The overall condition chart is primarily related to physical and emotional states. The social support chart is a subjective assessment of support but does not relate to patient needs. The quality of life chart is the most general question of all. The committee believes that the relationships between function, health, and quality of life may be conceived as concentric circles with a core being functional status, a surrounding circle that of health, and it is in turn surrounded by quality of life. Perhaps an outer circle might be labeled 'future." The several charts relate to these concentric circles as follows: physical condition, emotional condition, daily work, and social activities belong under function; pain, overall condition, and social support are part of health, which is the second circle; and quality of life is part of the third circle. Additional elements of quality of life include the availability of food, water, and shelter, as well as others.

The committee considered each of the COOP charts in detail and how it may either meet or fail to meet the needs of the committee. For each of the charts suggestions were made for modifications and how these charts may relate to other measures of function.

1. Physical Condition

This chart measures function in absolute rather than relative terms. It is really a measure of physical fitness. It relates well to the RAND 10 and 25 item questionnaires which give additional detail on physical functioning. Thus those two instruments could be used in a hierarchical fashion if information from the physical condition chart is insufficient. This chart appears to be a poor measure of small motor skills and insufficient to fully assess the activities of daily living. As mentioned above it correlates well with the RAND scales and in addition to the Duke-UNC Health Profile. The issue of time frame (i.e. During the last 4 weeks) which involved the other charts as well was discussed. Several time frames were suggested which included 4 weeks, 2 weeks, 1 week, 1 day and even 6 months. The time frame issue relates both to frequency of patient visits as well as patient's ability to recall health events. There was much support for using the 1 day or current time frame so that this chart would be introduced by a statement that said, "What is the most strenuous level of physical activity that you can do for at least 2 minutes?"

Additional changes recommended were to use a single set of pictures rather than a dual set and to simplify the illustrations, perhaps with stick drawings rather than dough-boy type drawings.

It was also noted that both physician and patient ratings may be useful, as well as both patient and health provider administration. It may be useful to have a place on the chart to designate who has done the rating and how the charts were administered. The committee also noted that the five categories were not equi-distant in terms of physical fitness and that these charts were not suitable for children. The committee did recommend retention of a five point scale for this chart as well as for all of the others. Lastly, there was the question of retitling this chart to Physical Fitness rather than Physical Condition.

2. Emotional Condition

This chart might very well be retitled "Feelings." It is noted that cognitive ability and issues of control of one's life were missing from this category of function. It was suggested that a group of second level instruments might include a mini-mental assessment for cognitive skills and a depression scale for patients with disturbed feelings. For this chart, too, there was discussion about time frame and also changing the type of drawings. A simple circle with changes of the mouth from a big smile to a big frown was suggested as a possible alternate.

3. Daily Work

It was noted that the word *work* may by difficult to translate into the several languages and may have different meanings within the several countries. It was noted too that this is a relative scale rather than one that is absolute and that there is an expanded instrument to measure this aspect of function produced by the RAND Corporation which interdigitates nicely with this chart. Daily activities or daily tasks might be more accurate titles although semi-literate persons may have more difficulty in understanding those meanings.

4. Social Activities

This scale generated considerable discussion. Some felt that social activities were not really a part of function. Others felt that there would be severe problems with translation of this chart and that it may be linked to daily work. The committee finally recommended that this chart be eliminated as a core chart since it correlates quite well with the first three charts and therefore may be superfluous. It may be used at a second level of administration rather than as a core chart.

5. Pain

It was noted that this chart is related to severity of disease. In addition there are other pain scales available such as a visual analog scale and the McGill Melzack pain questionnaire.

6. Change in Condition

This chart differs from the other in that a score of three indicates no change and for both improvement and getting worse there are only two levels available. Thus, it may be useful to add additional ranks. The committee felt that this scale required validation using both Dutch and United States data, and that the issue of appropriate time for reassessment was uncertain. There may be a lack of sensitivity in the use of this scale. In addition the illustrations might be improved.

7. Overall Condition

For this chart an alternate way of phrasing the question might be, "Overall how would you rate your health?" since it was noted that this chart is more a measure of health rather than of function.

8. Social Support

The committee felt that this chart, too, may be a secondary scale to be used if daily work is impaired. It was believed that the chart asks hypothetical questions and to some extent covers dependency, resources, and patients' fragility. It was noted that a dependency scale might be a very useful addition to the charts. Most of the committee members felt that this chart should be eliminated and that there was a need for another chart containing one item that would clearly define the essential components of social function. It was felt that the two charts on social issues, that is social support and social activities, did not measure social function.

9. Quality of Life

There was agreement that this chart should be eliminated from the core charts but it could be used for special purposes.

There are other aspects of function for which assessment is desirable. These are:

1. Communication (i.e. vision, speech, and hearing).
2. Coping ability. Can patients complete tasks? What is their level of optimism? What strategies have they adopted for coping? Are they able to relax?
3. Basic health needs. These encompass availability of water, food, and shelter, especially in underdeveloped countries.
4. Measurement of dependency.

An international version of the COOP charts are planned and in preparation. An international field test will follow.

Jack Froom
Chairman

Contents

Contributors

M. Baker, M.D.
Family Practice Group, Pocatello, ID, USA

John Barrand, L.M.S.S.A., D.A., F.R.A.C.G.P., M.H.P.E.D.
Department of Community Medicine, University of Sydney, Sydney, Australia

Bent Guttorm Bentsen, M.D.
Department of Community Medicine and General Practice, University of Trondheim, Trondheim, Norway

Niels Bentzen, M.D.
Department of General Practice, Institute of Community Health, Odense University, Odense, Denmark

W.J.H.M. van den Bosch, M.D.
Department of General Practice/Family Medicine, University of Nijmegen, Nijmegen, The Netherlands

Charles Bridges-Webb, M.D.
Division of Family Medicine, University of Sydney, Sydney, Australia

Terkel Christiansen, M.Sc.
Department of Economics, Odense University, Odense, Denmark

Richard T. Connis, Ph.D.
Department of Health Services, School of Public Health and Community Medicine, University of Washington, Seattle, WA, USA

Jan Craenen, M.D.
Department of General Practice, Catholic University of Leuven, Leuven, Belgium

Maria-Bernadette De Munter, M.D.
Department of General Practice, Catholic University of Leuven, Leuven, Belgium

Luc Dessers, M.D.
Department of General Practice, Catholic University of Leuven, Leuven, Belgium

R. Wayne Elford, M.D.
Department of Family Medicine, University of Calgary, Calgary, Alberta, Canada

Jack Froom, M.D.
Department of Family Medicine, State University of New York at Stony Brook, Health Sciences Center, Stony Brook, NY, USA

Michael J. Gordon, Ph.D.
Department of Family Medicine, School of Medicine, University of Washington, Seattle, WA, USA

Kristien Haepers, M.D.
Department of General Practice, Catholic University of Leuven, Leuven, Belgium

Ron D. Hays, Ph.D.
Behavioral Sciences Department, The RAND Corporation, Santa Monica, CA, USA

Jan Heyrman, M.D.
Department of General Practice, Catholic University of Leuven, Leuven, Belgium

Adam Keller, M.P.H.
Dartmouth COOP Project, Department of Community and Family Medicine, Dartmouth Medical School, Hanover, NH, USA

John W. Kirk, M.D.
The Dartmouth COOP Project, Department of Community and Family Medicine, Dartmouth Medical School, Hanover, NH, USA

Henk Lamberts, M.D., Ph.D.
Department of Family Medicine, University of Amsterdam, Amsterdam, The Netherlands

Jeanne M. Landgraf, M.A.
The Dartmouth COOP Project, Department of Community and Family Medicine, Dartmouth Medical School, Hanover, NH, USA

J.E. Liljenquist, M.D.
Private Practice, Idaho Falls, ID, USA

R.S. Mecklenberg, M.D.
Section of Endocrinology and Metabolism, Mason Clinic, Seattle, WA, USA

Betty Meyboom-de Jong, M.D., Ph.D.
Department of Family Medicine, University of Groningen, Groningen, The Netherlands

Mohib H. Mirza M.B.B.S., B.Sc., D.M.R.E., E.C.H.
College of Family Medicine, Punjab, Lahore, Pakistan

Eugene C. Nelson, Ph.D.
Director, Quality of Care Research, Hospital Corporation of America, Nashville, TN, USA

Kjeld Møller Pedersen, M.Sc.
Health Department, Vejle County Hospital, Vejle, Denmark

Tim B. Rogers, Ph.D.
Department of Psychology, University of Calgary, Calgary, Alberta, Canada

Hirosada Shigemoto, M.D.
Shigemoto Medical Clinic, Okayama, Japan

R.J.A. Smith, M.Sc.
Department of Family Medicine, State University of Groningen, Groningen, The Netherlands

A.J.A. Smits, M.D.
Department of General Practice/Family Medicine, University of Nijmegen, Nijmegen, The Netherlands

J.W. Stephens, M.D.
Portland Diabetes Center, Portland, OR, USA

Anita L. Stewart, Ph.D.
Institute of Health and Aging, University of California San Francisco, San Francisco, CA, USA

Tom R. Taylor, M.D., Ph.D.
Department of Family Medicine, School of Medicine, University of Washington, Seattle, WA, USA

Chris van Weel, M.D., Ph.D., Prof.
Department of General Practice/Family Medicine, University of Nijmegen, Nijmegen, The Netherlands

John H. Wasson, M.D.
The Dartmouth COOP Project, Department of Community and Family Medicine, Dartmouth Medical School, Hanover, NH, USA

S. Rae West, M.B.Ch.B.
Division of General Practice, School of Medicine, University of Auckland, Auckland, New Zealand

Robert C. Westbury, M.D. (Cantab.)
Family Physician, Calgary, Alberta, Canada

Michael Zubkoff, Ph.D.
Dartmouth COOP Project, Department of Community and Family Medicine, Dartmouth Medical School, Hanover, NH, USA

The WONCA Classification Committee

Dr. Jack Froom, Chairman	USA
Dr. Charles Bridges-Webb	Australia
Prof. Dr. Jan Heyrman	Belgium
Dr. Robert C. Westbury	Canada
Dr. Niels Bentzen	Denmark
Dr. A.K. Coates	England
Dr. Erik Hagman	Finland
Dr. Irene F. Osmund	Hong Kong
Dr. Bijon Chakraborty	India
Dr. Philip Sive	Israel
Dr. Hirosada Shigemoto	Japan
Dr. Bang Bu Youn	Korea
Dr. Kumar Rajakumar	Malaysia
Dr. Henk Lamberts	The Netherlands
Dr. S. Rae West	New Zealand
Dr. S.E. Mbanefo	Nigeria
Dr. Bent Guttorm Bentsen	Norway
Dr. Mohib H. Mirza	Pakistan
Dr. Primitivo D. Chua	Philipines
Dr. Eduardo Mendes	Portugal
Dr. Bill Dodd	Saudi Arabia
Dr. W.M. Patterson	Scotland
Dr. Paul Chan	Singapore
Dr. Dennis Aloysius	Sri Lanka
Dr. Britt-Gerd Malmberg	Sweden
Dr. Gisela Fischer	West Germany
Dr. Maurice Wood	USA

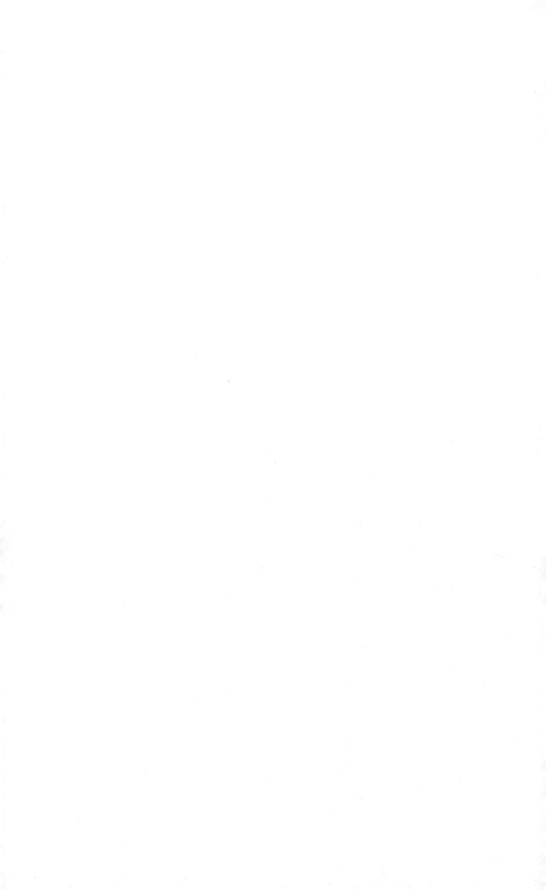

Part I   Psychometric Issues

1
Psychometric Considerations in Functional Status Instruments

A.L. STEWART

Psychometrics is simply about measurement. Good measures of the variables being studied are essential to assure that the questions of interest can be answered. The adequacy of measures can be judged in terms of their variability, reliability, validity (including response bias), sensitivity, practicality, and interpretability.* These features of good measures will be described here as they apply to measures of functional status in clinical settings. The advantages of multiitem measures over single-item measures are reviewed, and a few suggestions are made regarding the evaluation of the clinical utility of the measures.

The goal of the Classification Committee of WONCA is to select a set of measures of functional status (including measures of well-being) that can be used and understood by ordinary family doctors in their practices anywhere in the world. Before proceeding, it is important to clarify two quite distinct uses of such measures in clinical settings:

1. For research purposes, to build a database of information on functional status that can be linked with treatment and diagnostic information, to determine which treatments are better, and to determine the effects of various conditions.
2. For clinical purposes, to aid in the discovery of previously undiagnosed conditions, to facilitate a clinical decision, to provide information on

Paper presented at the workshop on functional status measurement in primary care, sponsored by the Classification Committee of WONCA (the World Organization of National Colleges, Academies and Academic Associations of General Practitioners/Family Physicians), Calgary, Alberta, Canada, October, 1988.

This invited presentation was to inform primary care physicians about basic psychometric principles and how they apply to the selection of measures of functional status and well-being for use in primary care practice.

*There are many good sources of information on psychometric principles and characteristics of good measures: for example, Guilford, 1954 (1); Nunnally, 1978 (2); McDowell and Newell, 1987 (3); Bergner and Rothman, 1987 (4); Ware, Brook, Davies-Avery, et al., 1980 (5).

changes in functioning of the individual patient to help monitor treatment effects, and to improve communication about the effects of health problems and their treatments.

These two basic purposes have different requirements in terms of the necessary properties of the measures. These requirements will be discussed in the sections below.

Variability and Distribution of Responses

Good variability means that the scores on a particular sample are spread out over the full range of the measure and that the distribution of the scores is roughly normal. The most common problem of variability in functional status measures is skewness, which means that the scores are mostly at one end of the scale. This usually occurs because people tend to be fairly functional, although many measures focus on the dysfunctional end of the scale. For example, in one application of the Nottingham Health Profile over half of the respondents scored zero (perfectly healthy) on each of the six measures (6).

Even if a measure varies greatly within one population, it might not within another. The Katz activities of daily living (ADL) index (7, 8) is a good example of this. It rates people in terms of several self-care activities, such as bathing and feeding. In the institutional settings in which the ADL was developed, patients received scores over the full range of activities, and decisions could be made based on the different scores. But if the scale is administered to ambulatory patients, nearly all the patients will get a perfect score; thus the scale is not as useful.

The distribution of measures is important because many statistical techniques are based on the assumption that variables are somewhat normally distributed. However, many commonly used measures of functional status are truly skewed (i.e., they reflect the true state of the population). Nevertheless, when a measure is very skewed, the problem can sometimes be corrected by adding questions that detect less serious problems.

Error in Measures

Before explaining reliability and validity, some background on the nature of error in measures would be useful. An observed score or a set of scores can be considered to have three components:

Observed score	=	True score	+	Systematic error	+	Random error

The true score is hypothetical—it refers to the actual amount of the attribute being measured. For example, the true score could be the person's true temperature.

There are three potential sources of error: the subject studied, the observer (if there is one), and the instrument used.

Systematic error is error in the observed score that is consistent; hence it is referred to as bias. For example, if a thermometer is miscalibrated, it may consistently register temperature that is lower than the true temperature (an instrument bias) or some people may consistently underreport their emotional problems (a subject bias).

Random error refers to an inconsistent error in the observed score, that is, the observed score may sometimes be higher and sometimes be lower than the true score. For example, a nurse may sometimes read the thermometer slightly high and sometimes slightly low because it is hard to read (an observer source of random error). If I ask a patient how many days during the past month he felt depressed, he might sometimes slightly overestimate and sometimes slightly underestimate, simply because he does not precisely know (a subject source of random error).

Good measurement involves increasing the amount of true score in the measure and decreasing the amount of error. There are ways to do this and ways to check to see if it has been done. Just as a thermometer can be calibrated to be more accurate, there are ways to design questions about functioning and well-being to minimize random error and bias (see, for example, reference 9).

Reliability

Reliability refers to the extent to which a score is free of random error. Some general synonyms for reliability are consistency, reproducibility, and repeatability. Hypothetically, it is the extent to which the same score would be obtained again using the same measuring instrument under the same conditions. To determine the level of cholesterol in a blood sample, the reliability of the determination is the extent to which the same level is obtained in subsequent determinations on aliquots of the same blood sample. If different levels are obtained, random error is occurring. Systematic error does not affect reliability; because it errs systematically (consistently in the same direction), it is reliable. Systematic error does affect validity, as will be seen below. Reliability is usually expressed as a coefficient from 0.00 to 1.00, with perfect reliability being 1.00

Why Is Reliability Important?

Adequate reliability is a prerequisite to using a score for any purpose (see, for example, reference 10). To the extent that a score is unreliable, the true score is obscured by error (or noise). Assume you are trying to determine if one treatment results in less fatigue than another one, and that one of the treatments really does. If the measure of fatigue is unreliable, when the two treatment groups are compared, the error in the score will be so high that the true difference is obscured. Put another way, the reliability of a measure limits the degree of validity (true score) that is possible. More technically, the correlation between two measures can never exceed the square root of the product of the measures' reliability (2). Thus, if both measures have a reliability of 0.70, their correlation, in theory, is limited to 0.70 (instead of 1.0, which in theory indicates a perfect correlation). This means that when a measure is not reliable, the actual relationship of that concept to other concepts cannot be known.

How Is Reliability Determined?

Table 1.1 presents a summary of the four most common types of reliability— internal consistency, test–retest, interrater, and the coefficient of reproducibility. The internal-consistency approach yields a reliability coefficient, sometimes called coefficient Alpha or Cronbach's Alpha (11) and is sometimes abbreviated r_{tt}. Internal-consistency reliability is used only for multiitem Likert scales, which are derived by adding together several items that have a similar response scale. For example, a Likert scale might consist of the addition of three questions that ask how often the person feels depressed, feels blue, and feels sad, all of which have the same response scale (1, often; 2, sometimes; 3, occasionally; 4, never). More information on Likert scales is presented below. The reliability coefficient is a function of two properties of scale items: (i) the extent to which the items have something in common, otherwise known as item homogeneity and (ii) the number of items in the scale. Reliability is increased when either property increases. Values of 0.50 or greater are considered evidence of adequate internal-consistency reliability; values between 0.70 and 0.90 are optimal.

Test–retest reliability can be used for single item measures as well as for multiitem scales. In test–retest reliability, the same questions are asked of the same group of people at two points in time and a correlation between the two tests is computed. The time between the test and the retest must be short enough so that substantial change in the attribute being measured is unlikely, yet long enough so that respondents will not remember their previous responses. If a change has occurred, the true reliability will be underestimated, and if respondents remember their previous responses, the true reliability will be overestimated (12, 13). As the time between the first measure and the second measure is increased, the coefficient may indicate the stability of the concept rather than the reliability of the test. This is truer for attributes that tend to change over time (e.g., health) than for those that tend to be relatively stable (e.g., attitudes, beliefs).

Interrater reliability refers to the consistency with which different raters or observers watching or rating the same person on an attribute simultaneously agree with one another (4). For example, the New York Heart Association

TABLE 1.1. Overview of most common types of reliability.

Type of reliability	Definition/explanation	Appropriate for:
Internal consistency (Coefficient Alpha, r_{tt})	The extent to which all items in the scale measure the same underlying concept, or the convergence of the items on the concept being measured; r_{tt} increases as the items become more homogeneous or similar and as the number of items increases	Multi-item (Likert) scales (see text)
Test–retest	The extent to which repeat administrations of the same measure are consistent; expressed as the correlation of the same measure administered at Time 1 and Time 2. The appropriate time difference depends on the nature of the measure and should be short enough so that the concept has not changed and long enough so that the respondent cannot easily recall his or her first response	All types of measures
Interrater	The extent to which one observer's rating of something is consistent with another observer's rating. Expressed as the correlation between the score or rating of one observer with that of another observer on the same person	Observer-rated measures
Coefficient of reproducibility (CR)	Reflects the extent to which a person's item responses can be predicted from knowledge of their (Guttman) scale score	Guttman scales (see text)

measure of disease severity requires that a physician rate the patient. A test of interrater reliability would involve correlating scores rated by one physician with scores rated by another. Again, the two raters would need to rate the person within an appropriate time frame to assure that the attribute being measured had not changed. Interrater reliability standards range from 0.80 to 1.00 (4).

The coefficient of reproducibility (CR) reflects the extent to which a Guttman (cumulative) scale score allows one to know precisely the pattern of response on each individual question from which the Guttman scale was derived. A cumulative or Guttman scale is one in which people respond to a series of yes or no items, each in turn reflecting a slightly more severe condition or more serious opinion. For example, a person would state whether they could walk with no difficulty: (i) one block, (ii) several blocks, or (iii) one mile. The scale score is the number of yes responses. Because of the ordered severity of items, a score of 1 would indicate that the person could walk a block but could not walk either several blocks or a mile. The CR also reflects reliability in the internal-consistency sense (5). A high CR indicates both reliability and reproducibility; values of 0.90 or greater are considered to indicate both (14, 15).

Acceptable Levels of Reliability

Of course, nearly all measures of everything contain some random error. The issue is what level of error is acceptable. The acceptable level of random error (or the acceptable reliability) depends on the use of the measure. To assess an individual patient on a clinical measure to determine whether to begin an expensive or unpleasant treatment regimen, the reliability criterion should be very high. Indeed, as Nunnally (2) points out, it is frightening to think that any measurement error is permitted in such situations. In applied settings in which important decisions are made with respect to specific scores, Nunnally recommends reliabilities of at least 0.90 and preferably 0.95. However, if the measure is intended only as a starting point for a discussion about potential functional status problems, such high reliabilities are not as critical.

For purposes of research in which decisions are made about relationships among variables within an entire sample (sometimes referred to as group comparisons), reliability can be lower. The accepted standard has been that 0.50 is adequate for group comparisons (16). The reason for this is that the random error will tend to average out across people when the sample is large.

Testing Reliability for Disadvantaged Groups

Reliability tends to be poorer in more disadvantaged groups such as people with little education (5, 17) and possibly the very old. This is probably because such people have more difficulty in reading and understanding questions or are less familiar with questionnaire procedures. If comparisons are to be made on outcome measures across groups that differ in these characteristics, it is important to test reliability separately in these groups, to assure that minimum standards are met for each group.

Validity

Validity refers to the extent to which a measure actually measures what we want it to and does not measure what we do not want it to. It can be thought of as the extent of true score in the measure.

The types of validity referred to in the literature include face, content, construct, discriminant, convergent, predictive, concurrent, criterion, known-groups, incremental, and probably others. This array of terms is confusing and their definitions are not always consistent. A taxonomy of the most common validity terms is presented in Table 1.2, which is based on the two

TABLE 1.2. Overview of types of validity.

Type of validity	Definition and examples
Content Validity	Are All Relevant Concepts Represented in the Measure or Set of Measures?
Content validity of a battery or collection of several measures	Are all important aspects of functioning and well-being represented in the set of health measures?
Content validity of a single multiitem scale	Are all aspects of the definition of the concept being measured represented in the scale? Does the label adequately represent the items in the scale?
Face validity	Do the items in the scale appear to measure the concept being measured?
Criterion-Related Validity	Does the Measure Correlate Highly with the "Gold Standard" Measure of That Concept?
Criterion validity	Does a new measure of depressive disorder correlate with the gold standard measure [e.g., Diagnostic Interview Schedule of the DSM-III (19)]?
Criterion-related validity	Does a short-form measure of emotional status have a high correlation with a validated, long-form measure of emotional status?
Predictive validity	Do scores on a measure of health perceptions predict whether people use any health services in the following year, or an unfavorable clinical outcome?
Construct Validity	Do the Measures Correlate with Measures of Other Variables in Hypothesized Ways?
Convergent validity	Does a measure of pain intensity correlate with a measure of the effects of pain?
Discriminant validity	Does a measure of physical functioning have a lower correlation with a measure of mental health than with a measure of mobility?
Multitrait–multimethod approach	Does a self-reported measure of depression have a higher correlation with an observer rating of depression than with a self-reported measure of anxiety?
Known-groups validity	Is the mean health perceptions score significantly lower for a group of patients than for a general population sample?
Studies of Bias	Are Scores Systematically Lower or Higher due to Response Bias?
	Are scores of social functioning significantly correlated with a measure of socially desirable responding?

most commonly cited classification schemes.* Three basic types of validity are content validity, criterion-related validity, and construct validity, each of which are defined below. One other important validity issue that does not fall neatly into one of these categories is whether there are sources of bias or systematic error in the scores.

Validation involves the convergence of information from many sources; thus it is an "unending" process of compiling empirical evidence (2). That is, each piece of evidence for the validity of a measure or a set of measures provides added support for the validity of a measure, but there is no one point at which a measure is considered valid. Therefore, the validation of health measures cannot be thoroughly determined in a single study.

A comprehensive or complete evaluation of validity for a measure of functional status requires multiple sources of data (e.g., self-report, physician report, independent clinical assessment) and longitudinal data to determine the ability of the measures to predict subsequent health and utilization. In addition, it is important to test the validity in different population groups (e.g., general populations, patients with heart disease, patients with depression).

Because a specific health measure may be used for different purposes, its validity may need to be determined separately for each purpose. A health measure that is valid for one purpose will not necessarily be valid for another (20). For example, if a measure is needed to identify patients at risk for some future event, its validity needs to be determined in terms of its ability to do just that. If measures are to be used to evaluate the quality of care, some of the most important validity tests should be in terms of whether the measures are able to detect known differences in the quality of care. This may sound somewhat circular, but is not as bad as it sounds. As a validation study, this requires that we can identify good and poor quality of care or define a continuum ranging from poor to good. Once such a known quality of care measure is available, we can test hypotheses about the relationship of known quality of care to these outcomes.

Content Validity

Content validity is a qualitative approach to determining validity. A look at the concepts that are represented in a battery of health measures, or a look at the content of the items included in a particular scale, is the essence of this approach. Content validity thus refers to how well a specified domain of content is sampled (2). To determine content validation requires a definitional standard against which the measures or items are being compared.

To determine the content validity of a *particular* measure, the items can be

---

*The American Psychological Association, the American Educational Research Association, and the National Council on Measurement in Education (18) and Nunnally (2).

reviewed to see if all aspects of standard definitions of that concept are represented. For example, a measure of physical functioning should include items referring to walking, running, bending, lifting, carrying things, climbing stairs, and walking uphill, all of which are fairly commonly agreed-upon components of physical functioning.

To determine the content validity of a *battery* of measures, for example, the list of concepts can be compared against some complete conceptual framework of all possible functioning concepts. Some efforts to provide this definitional framework have been made (see, for example, references 21–24). This type of validation requires confidence in the definitional standard.

Content validity is an important consideration during the construction and development of measures (2, 18). That is, items in a scale, or scales in a battery, should be selected at the outset to assure content validity.

Face validity is a special type of content validity that focuses on the extent to which each item in a measure appears to measure that which it purports to. Face validity is the "commonsense" part of content validity, that which assures that the items are to the point.

Criterion-Related Validity

Criterion validity. Clinicians are probably more familiar with criterion approaches to validity. If a reasonably good clinical measure is available, such as cholesterol level or blood pressure readings, and a new measure is proposed that is cheaper or simpler, or perhaps can be used by the patient at home, the new measure should be tested against the "gold standard," which becomes the criterion. A high correlation of the new measure with the criterion measure is considered to be evidence of validity.

Criterion-related validity. In assessing functioning and well-being, there are no gold standard criterion measures for comparison. However, there are some situations in which scores on the measure being validated are used to predict some criterion. For example, we can compare a newer, very short measure of functioning against a longer, well-validated measure of functioning, which becomes the criterion. Because it is not a true criterion, the term criterion related has been adopted.

Clinicians frequently require evidence that measures of functioning and well-being correlate with clinical measures, as if a clinical measure represented the criterion. Although such a correlation might be considered evidence of construct validity, clinical measures are not criteria against which generic measures should be compared (see below).

Predictive validity. When a measure is to be used to predict some behavior or event that is external to the measure itself, the behavior or event is referred to as the *criterion* and the analysis is called *predictive validity* (2). The predicted behavior or event can be at the same point in time (*concurrent validity*) or in the future. The prediction can be made in terms of group membership (e.g., any hospitalizations) or in terms of a continuous measure (e.g., expenditures for health care; subsequent disease severity or functional status). In general, the higher the correlation the better.

If measures are to be used for the purpose of identifying patients who are likely to use a lot of health care services, to identify patients at risk of poor health in the future (in greater need of care), or to identify patients most likely to respond to a treatment, then the validity of the measures must be determined in terms of their ability to predict these variables. In these cases, the outcome to be predicted becomes a true criterion, and criterion validity studies are necessary.

Construct Validity

The basic issue in studies of construct validity is whether the health measures relate to other measures in ways consistent with plausible hypotheses. Thus, hypotheses are stated regarding the direction (and sometimes the strength) of relationships between the measure being validated and measures of other variables, based on theory and on reported findings. Correlations are then examined to see if the hypothesized patterns are confirmed (2, 25). Validity is supported when the observed correlations conform to the hypotheses. When the hypothesized relationships are not observed, and the theory is well founded, the validity should be questioned. It is important that hypotheses be firmly grounded in theory. If the logic of the hypotheses is poorly thought through, a null finding might be taken as an indication of poor validity when in fact it reflects a true situation (3). For example, in early validity studies of measures of functioning and well-being, the correlation of the measures with age was tested, and a positive correlation (older people experience poorer functioning and well-being) was taken as a sign of validity. Although this may be true of such variables as physical functioning, it is not necessarily true for all variables (e.g., it does not seem to be true for emotional status). Thus, the lack of a correlation of age and emotional status reflects a true state rather than poor validity.

It is as important to test hypotheses about relationships that should not occur as well as those that should. This principle is easier to understand when considering classification variables, such as the presence or absence of something (as in many diagnostic tests). For example, the test for Down's syndrome should detect it when it is truly present (sensitivity). Just as important is that the test not detect Down's syndrome if it is not present (specificity). Thus, a valid test is one that has high sensitivity and specificity. The application of this principle to more continuous functional status measures is slightly more complicated, but the principle is the same.

There is a good example of the validity of depression measures that illustrates the concept of construct validity. Many measures of depression used in mental health research include questions about feeling sad, tired, worth-less, and lacking an appetite. These aspects of depression are included in a well-known depression measure, the Beck Depression Inventory (26). However, the more somatic items (e.g., feeling tired, loss of appetite) may also be symptoms of some physical problem. Thus, this measure may not be a valid depression measure for patients of primary care physicians because it contains information on both depression and physical health (see, for example, references 27 and 28). The measure does indeed detect depression, that is, it is sensitive to depression (it has convergent validity). However, it detects other things as well such physical health problems, that is, it is not specific to depression (it lacks discriminant validity).

The "art" in designing good construct validity studies is to identify key concepts for which good hypotheses can be stated and to include good measures of these in the validity studies. The correlation of health measures with clinical status measures usually falls within this type of evaluation—that is, we can hypothesize that certain measures of functioning or well-being would correlate with certain clinical measures. In this case, the clinical measures are not considered as criteria but rather as constructs that the health measures should be related to. It is often said that a criterion for good measures of functioning or well-being is that the measures should be sensitive to changes in clinical status. In terms of validity, a measure of functioning should be related to a measure of clinical status if such a relationship can be hypothesized in advance. But not all changes in clinical status will affect functioning, and when no relationship is found, it does not mean the measure is not good. For example, we expect to see a decline in physical functioning when a person's arthritis becomes more severe. But we would not expect to see a decline in physical functioning when blood pressure rises.

Convergent validity. Convergent validity is like sensitivity. It means that a measure should correlate with other measures of the same concept. For example, one could test the relationship between two measures of the same concept using different methods (e.g., physical functioning based on self-report and physical functioning rated by an observer). An appropriate indicator of convergent validity is the correlation coefficient. Although a correlation of 0.40 is considered to be a substantial validity coefficient (29), generally the higher the correlation, the better the validity.

Discriminant validity. Discriminant validity is like specificity. It means that a measure should not be related to measures of other concepts it is not supposed to relate to. For example, a measure of physical functioning would not be expected to be highly related to a measure of depression or of loneliness. Because all health measures are related to one another to some extent, we do not look for zero correlations in determining discriminant validity. Instead, we look for correlations that are lower than the convergent validity correlations. That is, we determine whether measures correlate lower with measures they are not expected to be related to than they do with measures they are expected to be related to. For this reason, the term *convergent/discriminant validity* is more often used.

Multitrait–multimethod approach. When more than one method has been used to collect data on a particular variable (for example, self-report and observer rating), a multitrait–multimethod approach can be used (30). The essence of this approach is to test whether two measures of the same concept using different methods correlate more highly than do two measures of different concepts using the same method.

Known-groups validity. Known-groups validity is a type of construct validity that involves comparing mean scores on a health measure across groups known to differ in the concept being validated (31). For example, perceived health should be poorer in groups with a more severe disease (e.g., heart disease, cancer) than in those with a less severe disease (e.g., back problems, hypertension). In the Medical Outcomes Study, we confirmed that mean functioning and well-being scores were consistently poorer in a patient sample than in a general population—a known-groups validity study of our short-form health survey (32). To determine validity, it is important for us to know that the defined groups clearly differ in the concept or construct being tested. If the logic is poor, a finding of no difference might be taken to indicate poor validity when in fact it reflects a true situation (3).

Bias: Threats to Validity

There are two main sources of systematic error that sometimes go hand in hand with self-reported methods: socially desirable response set (SDRS), and acquiescent response set. These are referred to as response bias.

Socially Desirable Response Set

People often answer questions so as to represent themselves favorably. This is called *socially desirable responding* and is one of the most important sources of response bias in self-report research. Socially desirable responding affects the validity of self-reports because it leads to underreporting of socially undesirable characteristics or behavior and to overreporting of socially desirable ones (2).

There are two basic approaches to handling SDRS: minimizing its occurrence in the design of the questions asked and the methods used for collecting the information, and measuring it so its effects can be evaluated and controlled for.

By selecting appropriate methods for measuring those characteristics most likely to be susceptible to socially desirable responding, we can minimize its occurrence in these measures. For example, Dillman (33) has reported that SDRS tends to be less problematic in mail surveys than it is in telephone and face-to-face interviews (pp. 62–63). Accurate information on people's weight is more likely to be obtained by asking people to write their weight down on a questionnaire than if some thin person asks them face to face how much they weigh.

Socially desirable responding can also be minimized by writing questions that make it easy to make an "undesirable" response (34). If you ask patients if they are taking the medicine you prescribed, or sticking to the diet you recommended, you will probably get some socially desirable responding. If instead you ask them what kind of problems they are having taking the medicine or sticking to the diet, you are leaving the door open for them to admit those problems.

Acquiescent Response Set

Some people have a tendency to agree with anything you ask. This accounts for the well-known phenomenon in public opinion polls that yield different results depending on how questions are worded. Acquiescence tends to occur more often when questions are ambiguous, lengthy, complicated, or otherwise difficult to understand, and it is more likely to occur in less educated people (35). It can thus be minimized by keeping questions simple, clear, and short. It can also be minimized by using several questions to measure each concept, some with favorable wording and some with unfavorable wording (e.g., do you have a lot of energy? Do you feel tired?). When these questions are summed into a scale, agreement acquiescence tends to cancel out.

Sensitivity of Scores

As noted earlier, clinicians are most familiar with the term *sensitivity* with respect to classification measures. A sensitive measure is one that detects a high proportion of true cases. For more continuous functional status and well-being measures, sensitivity has a slightly different meaning. Here we do not want to detect a case, rather, we want a measure to be sensitive to important changes in the true attribute being measured. For example, in measuring pain, the measure should discriminate between people with meaningful differences in actual pain (e.g., between those with no pain, mild pain, moderate pain, and severe pain). The extent to which important differences in actual pain are reflected in the measure is an indicator of the pain measure's sensitivity.

Sensitivity is one aspect of validity, but we need to use a more refined approach to determine it than is usually used in validity studies. We actually know less about the sensitivity of our various measures than we do about all the other qualities of measurement because our methods for evaluating sensitivity are not very sophisticated. We hope that, over the next few years, psychometricians will become more creative in this area.

Assume you want to know when a treatment strategy has actually reduced the pain of a group of patients. A pain measure is needed that is able to discriminate those changes in pain that are important. Table 1.3 illustrates a

TABLE 1.3. An illustration of the relative sensitivity of three pain measures.

True pain before and after optimal treatment and OK treatment:

Excruciating - - - - - - - - - - - X - - - - - - - - -X- - - - - - - - - X - - - - - - - No pain

	Before treatment	After OK treatment	After optimal treatment

Pain measure 1:

(1)	(2)	(3)
[a lot of pain][	some pain	][no pain]

Pain measure 2:

(1)	(2)	(3)	(4)	(5)
[very much][	quite a bit][	some	][a little][	no pain]

Pain measure 3:

Very much   No pain

[1][2][3][4][5][6][7][8][9][10]

hypothetical situation of a "true" change in pain due to two different treatments and how three hypothetical measures of pain might determine the true change.

Measure 1 is not sensitive enough to detect either change in the amount of pain—a score of 2 is obtained both before and after either treatment. Measure 2 may be sensitive enough to detect the change due to the optimal treatment but not sensitive enough to detect the change due to the OK treatment. However, we must assume that measure 2 is reliable. If there is random error such that people might have trouble knowing whether to report a 3 or a 4, the measure may not detect the true change. Measure 3 may be sensitive enough to either treatment, even if there is some random error.

Of course, this example is hypothetical, and so the true pain and the true change due to the best treatment can be presented. But it illustrates a principle that the more points along the scale that are meaningful, the more sensitive the measure will be to meaningful change.

The sensitivity of a measure is something to consider when the appropriate measures for a particular use are selected. To follow everyday patients in terms of the effects of reassurance or medicine or treatment, a measure should be chosen that focuses on the range of functioning and well-being when these effects are expected. If a treatment for angina is expected to improve patients' ability to walk around, so they can walk further, then a measure of ADL, which focuses on basic self-care in addition to walking, will not be sensitive with respect to being able to walk different distances.

Deyo and Patrick (36) discuss several issues on how to evaluate the sensitivity of scales to clinically meaningful changes. They note that scale scores should be stable in patients who do not change clinically and that the scores should be responsive to clinical changes. Deyo and Inui (37) and Deyo and Centor (38) present some excellent methods for determining the sensitivity of scale scores to clinical changes. For example, they compared scores on various dimensions of the Sickness Impact Profile (SIP) to clinical judgments of improvement or deterioration (37). They found that the SIP score became progressively worse relative to an evaluation of clinical severity rated by the doctor, which indicated its sensitivity to known clinical changes.

Advantages of Multiitem Measures

If it is important that measures be sensitive enough to detect important differences, and since we know very little about the nature of those differences, it is to our advantage to use measures that have enough scale levels to increase the probability of such sensitivity.

However, the number of levels that can be assessed using a single item is limited. If patients are asked to rate their pain on a scale from 1 to 100, it is tempting to conclude that this 100-point scale is extremely sensitive. But the problem now reverts back to one of reliability and validity. Apparently it is very difficult for anyone to discriminate more than about seven levels along any scale involving judgment. Miller (39) referred to this concept as the magic number 7 (plus or minus 2). He hypothesized that there is a limit on the number of units of information that can be processed at one time. This magical number apparently also applies to people's ability to discriminate between feelings (40). In any case, even though a scale from 1 to 100 is provided, most people will look at the line with all those numbers and unwittingly convert it to a line with about seven categories. They can perhaps accurately rate themselves within those seven, or possibly fewer, categories, but not likely more. Thus, a person who marks a 52 and a person who marks a 58 might look different, but they really are not different because both numbers fall within only one of the seven categories. For this reason, most survey questions have only five or six response choices.

Just how does one achieve all this sensitivity? This is where various scaling methods come into play; here several questions are asked on each concept and added together or combined in some way to obtain a more continuous score with many scale levels.

When responses to several questionnaire items are summed into a single-scale score, it is called a *summated* or a *Likert-type scale*. A simple example of a summated ratings scale will illustrate this method. Suppose you have two items—"How often during the last four weeks did you have a lot of energy?" and "How often during the last four weeks did you feel tired?"—each with the following response choices:

1. None of the time.
2. A little of the time.
3. Some of the time.
4. Most of the time.
5. All of the time.

A summated ratings (Likert) scale of these two items would involve first reversing the scores on the second item (1, All of the time, 2, Most of the time, etc.) to make a high score on both items refer to energy, and then adding the item scores together. The lowest possible score on this summated scale would be two (two minimum-item scores of one each) and the highest possible score would be ten (two maximum-item scores of five each). By doing this, we have automatically improved the variability of the score—we now have nine possible scale levels instead of just five. This increases the chance that the measure will be sensitive to important differences. Further, we have not required people to rate themselves using more than five categories.

The combination of several questions has several other advantages. The reliability of the final score is increased over that of any one of the questions. This occurs because of pooling or combining the "true score" portion that each of the items has in common, thus coming up with more true score.

The validity of the measure is improved by combining several questions, especially for such complex concepts as functional status and well-being. These concepts are often defined in terms of many things, and thus are difficult to measure using just one question. For example, physical functioning is defined in terms of walking, bending, lifting, stooping, and climbing stairs. The use of multiple items or questions allows one to "cast light at different angles" (35) (p. 47).

As an example, consider the construct of pain. You can ask people how intense it is when it occurs or how often they have it or how long it lasts when they have it. Thus, to measure the pain the person has had over a typical week adequately, you would want to take into account all of these things. The more aspects of the pain that your measure reflects, the more valid is the measure.

Certain kinds of systematic error are minimized when several items are combined. If people have a tendency to agree with your questions, by asking several positively worded questions and several negatively worded questions, any systematic tendency to agree is canceled out when the questions are combined.

Finally, if some item responses are missing, a score can still be estimated based on other items in the measure, thus reducing the amount of missing data on final scores.

The Interpretability of Scale Scores

For single-item measures with verbal response categories, the meaning of each score is quite clear. For example, the commonly used rating of health as excellent, very good, good, fair, or poor usually has scores from 1 to 5, and a score of 1 clearly means excellent health. However, when several items are combined into a Likert-type score, scores are possible over a broad range of numbers, and a particular score has no inherent meaning. This is one advantage of single-item measures over multiitem measures.

There are two issues regarding the interpretability of scores: (i) the meaning of particular score values and (ii) the meaning of differences in score values (between groups or between individuals) or of changes in score values over time.

Meaning of Score Values

We might ask: Using a six-item measure of physical functioning, what is the meaning of a score of 75?

First we need to know the possible range of scores or end points of the scale. We usually transform our measures to 0 to 100 scales, to facilitate this. This does not mean that we have 100 possible scale levels. It only means that we transpose the original end points of say 4 to 20 so that those with a 4 now have a 0, and those with 20 now have a 100, and the "in-between" scores are spread out proportionately between 0 and 100. This does not change the statistical properties of the score, it just makes it easier to remember the end points. We do this because when scales are of different lengths, the end points are always changing. So now we know that the score of 75 lies between 0 and 100.

Next we need to know what a high score means, or the direction of scoring. Does a high score mean better functioning or worse functioning? If 100 is the best functioning, 75 is about 75% of a perfect score. All tables in which any health score is presented are more useful if they contain information on the direction of scoring of the measures.

If the score of 75 is a score of an individual patient, you need to have some norms or standards against which to compare the score. When scores are developed in a general population or in some representative sample, the mean and the standard deviation of those samples become the norms against which scores of various subgroups can be compared. If you know, for example, that the mean physical functioning score for a general population is 85, and that the mean score for a representative patient sample is 75, you can interpret the score of an individual patient relative to these norms.

Meaning of Score Differences

Because we mainly use health measures to determine if various treatments or types of health care are effective, it is of more interest to understand the meaning of a difference in scores or a change over time. For example, What is the meaning of a five-point or a ten-point change in the score? Or a better question might be, What is the meaning of a difference of 0.1 standard deviation, or of 0.5 standard deviation? Does a five-point change in a pain measure reflect a change that is meaningful to the patient? Or is this not even a noticeable difference? Does a five-point change reflect what physicians would consider an optimal treatment effect? Or is much more relief possible?

This issue is closely related to the sensitivity of the scores, but it is distinct. Sensitivity pertains to whether the scores can detect important true differences in the concept being measured, or whether they can detect the effects of particular treatments. The issue of interpretability focuses more on just what a particular amount of change actually means to the patient or the doctor.

This has been called the calibration of measures or effect size analysis (29). Calibration involves documenting the meaning of differences in health scores by expressing them in terms that are clinically and socially relevant. An example of such an analysis is to determine the percent of patients who received mental health care whose scores on a psychological distress measure improved. Another example would be to examine the amount in a score resulting from the onset of a particular acute or chronic condition or a change associated with an especially effective therapy.

This is an area in which we know very little about most of the available measures of functioning and well-being. As we learn more about the meaning of changes in our scores, these measures will be more useful to clinicians in their everyday practices.

In the Health Insurance Experiment, a five point change (out of 100) in health perceptions was equivalent to the effect of knowing one has mild hypertension (41). The Medical Outcomes Study (MOS) has contributed some information on the meaning of some of the health scores by documenting the unique decrements in health due to each of nine chronic medical conditions. For example, we know that a nine-point difference on an MOS physical functioning score (scored from 0 to 100) is equivalent to the effect of having arthritis or back problems, controlling for other medical conditions (42). This type of information contributes to our understanding of the meaning of score differences and changes.

We could also examine the change in health scores associated with a known change in clinical status (e.g., the onset of a particular chronic condition or a change in severity). To document the meaning of score differences in relation to known clinical measures (e.g., blood pressure, use of health services) does not imply that these other measures are criteria against which the measures are being validated, as I have already mentioned. Rather, it is an attempt to translate the meaning of score differences into units that clinicians know, to facilitate their understanding of the scores. For example, Deyo and Inui (137) found that a seven-point decline in the SIP physical score was equal to a change from being able to do all usual activities to having discomfort or limited mobility of one or more joints on the Arthritis Rheumatoid Association functional classification.

However, a five-point difference at one end of the scale may not mean the same thing as a similar difference at the other end of the scale. That is, a five-point improvement at the severe end of the scale may mean far more to patients than a five-point improvement at the healthy end of the scale.

Studies such as these are badly needed to make measures more useful in clinical practice. With large sample sizes, it is relatively easy to obtain statistically significant differences in health scores, but it does not necessarily follow that the differences are meaningful.

Practicality/Feasibility

Administration and Burden

The best set of measures will be useless in everyday practice if they are difficult to use. That is, if the administration of the measures is going to disrupt the flow of patients, irritate the receptionist, and frustrate the patients, their use is not feasible in the office setting.

Social scientists are often criticized for not understanding how to fit their lengthy questionnaires into routine office practice. However, doctors and nurses often overestimate the extent to which patients will feel put upon to answer personal questions about the ways in which their health problems are affecting their daily lives and feelings. Thus, the task is to develop our measures and methods such that they can be most easily absorbed into routine office practice and so that they do not unduly burden patients. This certainly can be achieved, but it requires the application of a great deal of creative energy.

Nelson and his colleagues can be commended for their work in trying to understand how their COOP chart measures affected office staff and clinicians (43, 44). They have learned a lot about how to work with clinicians in their offices, and they can provide us with a lot of expertise in how to do this with other types of measures.

In the MOS, over 20,000 questionnaires, which took an average of 9 minutes to complete, were obtained from patients at the time of an office visit to one of the MOS clinicians. The RAND survey group was able to determine how to do this without disrupting offices or annoying staff (45).

Clinicians and office staff should know that patients are often delighted to answer these questions—in some cases, no one ever asked them such questions before. This can make them feel important, useful, and pleased that someone is interested. In a study by Nelson et al. (43), 89% of patients reported enjoying answering the questions using the chart method.

Scoring and Presentation of Scores

Are the scores easy to derive and present to the clinicians? For research purposes, the collection of large amounts of information is not a problem because it is coded, scored, and analyzed in batches, usually by computer. Plenty of time can be taken to summarize scores and present them in ways to facilitate their understanding.

For purposes of using the scores during an office visit, however, this is more of a problem. A method is needed to allow the information to be collected from the patient and put into the chart in an interpretable form before the doctor sees the patient. This means that about the only practical method is a short set of single questions, like the COOP charts. The scores for these can be interpreted without special scoring. For example, a 3 on the physical functioning chart means that the person can do moderate physical activities (but not heavy or very heavy activities).

As we have noted, if the score is going to be used as a basis for making clinical decisions or to monitor patients' progress over time, its reliability should be very high and it should be sensitive to the true changes that are occurring. We noted that multiitem measures are more likely to be highly reliable and sensitive. But to administer a longer set of questions to patients, score them, and present the score to the doctor is quite a challenge. Further, methods of graphically presenting the scores for optimal understanding by clinicians should be studied. The actual score should be presented in relation to some norm or standard (see, for example; references 46 and 47) and possibly, with suggestions or recommendations regarding treatment options (36).

We will probably see a surge in technological devices to do this, so should begin to think about how best to do it. With the increasing use of personal computers, patients will become more computer-wise and less averse to using a computer. A four-button, toylike device that can be used by patients to answer a series of questions, which is amazingly uncomputerlike and unintimidating, has been developed at the University of Chicago. It needs no cord at the time it is used, it can incorporate a variety of question sets, and when the patient is through, it can be plugged into a printer and the scores derived and printed out. Thus, we should not rule out the possibility of being able to use multiitem measures in assessing individual patients in office settings.

Clinical Utility

When we use such measures for research purposes, whether the measure is useful depends on the research questions being answered. This is an area that does not need further attention here. However, when measures are to be used by clinicians in their everyday practice, another issue must be dealt with: What is the usefulness to clinicians of knowing scores on these measures? It is increasingly being suggested that it is important to know patients' functional status (48–50), but it has yet to be demonstrated exactly how clinicians can make use of the information. Except in geriatric care, early efforts have indicated a lack of usefulness (see, for example, references 51–53; also cited in reference 36); thus, further work in this area is called for. At this stage in the implementation of these measures into everyday office practice, good methodological studies of the relative clinical utility of the different types of measures are needed.

There are several potential uses of such measures such as identifying functional problems that might lead to a new diagnosis, improving communication or creating more rapport between physicians and patients, and helping physicians make treatment decisions or decisions to refer patients for psychosocial help, and so forth. Why not study the extent to which various functional assessment batteries fulfill these potential functions?

Two basic approaches can be taken to addressing these questions. First, clinicians could be systematically surveyed regarding just what it is they would like to know about their patients' functioning and well-being. What is the relative usefulness of knowing about different aspects of people's lives? Is it more useful to learn about patients' physical functioning? Or how patients feel emotionally? Is it useful to know what a patient's general emotional state is? Or just the extent to which patients are upset about their health problems? Different functional status batteries include different types of information; thus, the selection of an appropriate battery depends on which types are desired. What will clinicians do with the information? Physicians may not want to know about problems they do not know how to treat (36).

A second approach would be to test the relative usefulness of various types of information and various ways of providing the information to clinicians empirically. For example, one could compare the number of new problems identified in a patient sample using the COOP charts and using another, longer-form battery. This comparison would take into account the relative sensitivities of the two batteries to new problems, as well as the practicality. If one measure were so impractical that patients couldn't complete it in time, or if physicians had trouble making use of the score, then even if it were more sensitive it would not help identify more problems.

Conclusions and Recommendations

The implementation of measures of functioning and well-being into medical practice is a revolution of sorts, and the Classification Committee of WONCA is at its forefront. Although the committee is eager to proceed with the selection of a battery for widespread implementation, I would urge consideration of several possible approaches in terms of their relative merits. Because different types of measures have different advantages and disadvantages, it is not easy to identify those best suited for individual purposes.

The main trade-off that needs to be studied regarding the use of these measures by clinicians in an office setting is between the use of single-item and multiitem measures. Single-item measures such as the COOP charts are more practical and interpretable, but multiitem measures may be much more sensitive to what it is the clinician wants to know and allow more complexity to be reflected in the measures, although implementation and interpretation are more difficult.

Rather than simply selecting a set of measures, I recommend considering several approaches and conducting a series of methodological studies as they are implemented. WONCA is in an ideal position to evaluate the different possibilities carefully and, eventually, recommend the best approach.

Acknowledgment. Samuel A. Bozzette, M.D. provided helpful comments on an earlier draft of this chapter.

References

1. Guilford JP. *Psychometric Methods*. New York, McGraw-Hill, 1954.
2. Nunnally JC. *Psychometric Theory*, ed 2. New York, McGraw-Hill, 1978.
3. McDowell IY, Newell C. *Measuring Health: A Guide to Rating Scales and Questionnaries*. New York, Oxford University Press, 1987.
4. Bergner M, Rothman ML. Health status measures: An overview and guide for selection. *Am Rev Public Health* 8:191–210, 1987.
5. Ware JE, Brook RH, Davies-Avery A, et al. *Conceptualization and Measurement of Health for Adults in the Health Insurance Study: Vol. I, Model of Health and Methodology*. Santa Monica, CA; The Rand Corp. (publication number R-1987/1-HEW), 1980.
6. Hunt SM, McKenna SP, McEwen J, Williams J, Papp E. The Nottingham Health Profile: Subjective health status and medical consultations. *Soc Sci Med* 15A:221–229, 1981.
7. Katz S, Ford AB, Moskowitz RW, Jackson BA, Jaffe MW. Studies of illness in the aged: The index of ADL. *JAMA* 185:914–919, 1963.
8. Katz S, Downs TD, Cash HR, Grotz RC. Progress in the developement of the Index of ADL. *The Gerontologist* Spring, 1970, pp. 20–30.
9. Bradburn NM, Sudman S, et al. *Improving Interview Method and Questionnaire Design*. San Francisco, Jossey-Bass Publishers, 1979.
10. Thorndike RL. Reliability. In Jackson DN, Messick S (eds). *Problems in Human Assessment*. New York, McGraw-Hill, 1967.
11. Cronbach LJ. Coefficient alpha and the internal structure of tests. *Psychometrika* 15:297–334, 1951.
12. Anastasi A. *Psychological Testing*, ed 4. New York, MacMillan, 1976.
13. Nachmias C, Nachmias D. *Research Methods in the Social Sciences*. London, St. Martins Press, 1981.
14. Edwards AL. *Techniques of Attitude Scale Construction*. New York, Appleton-Century-Crofts Inc., 1957.
15. Guttman LA. A basis for scaling qualitative data. *Am Sociol Rev* 9:139–150, 1944.
16. Helmstadter GC. *Principles of Psychological Measurement*. New York, Appleton-Century-Crofts, Inc., 1964.
17. Andrews FM. Construct validity and error components of survey measures: A structural modeling approach. *Pub Opin Quart* 48:409, 1984.
18. American Psychological Association. *Standards for Educational and Psychological Testing*. Washington, DC, American Psychological Association, 1985.
19. Robins LR, Helzer JE, Croughan J, Ratliff KS. National Institute of Mental Health Diagnostic Interview Schedule: Its history, characteristics, and vaildity. *Arch Gen Psychiatry* 38:381–389, 1981.
20. Ware JE, Brook RH, Davies AR, Lohr K. Choosing measures of health status for individuals in general populations. *Am J Pub Health* 71:620–625, 1981.
21. Ware JE. Standards for validating health measures: Definitions and content *J Chron Dis* 40:473–480, 1987.
22. Stewart AL. A framework of health indicators. In Stewart AL, Ware JE (eds). *Measuring Functional Status and Well-Being: The Medical Outcomes Study Approach* (Manuscript submitted for publication).
23. Bergner M. Measurement of health status. *Med Care* 23:696–704, 1985.

24. Gilson BS, Gilson JS, Bergner M, et al. The Sickness Impact Profile: Development of an outcome measure of health care. *Am J Pub Hlth* 65:1304–1310, 1975.
25. Cronbach LJ, Meehl PE. Construct validity in psychological tests. *Psych Bull* 52:281–302, 1955.
26. Beck AT, Ward CH, Mendelson M, et al. An inventory for measuring depression. *Arch Gen Psych* 4:53–63, 1961.
27. Koenig R, Levin SM, Brennan MJ. The emotional status of cancer patients as measured by a psychological test. *J Chron Dis* 20:923–930, 1967.
28. Silberfarb PM, Maurer LH, Crouthmel CS. Psychosocial aspects of neoplastic disease: I, Functional status of breast cancer patients during different treatment regimens. *Am J Psychia* 137:450–455, 1980.
29. Ware JE. Methodological considerations in the selection of health assessment procedures. In Wenger NK et al. (eds) *Assessment of quality of life in clinical trials of cardiovascular therapies.* New York: Le Jacq Publishing Inc., 1984.
30. Campbell DT, Fiske DW. Convergent and discriminant validation by the multitrait–multimethod matrix. *Psychol Bull* 56:81–105, 1959.
31. Kerlinger FN, Pedhazur EJ. *Multiple Regression in Behavioral Research.* New York: Holt, 1973.
32. Stewart AL, Hays RD, Ware JE. The MOS Short-Form General Health Survey: Reliability and validity in a patient population. *Med Care* 26:724–735, 1988.
33. Dillman DA. *Mail and Telephone Surveys: The Total Design Method.* New York, Wiley & Sons, 1978.
34. Edwards AL. *The measurement of personality traits by scales and inventories.* New York, Holt, Rinehart & Winston, 1970.
35. Converse JM, Presser S. *Survey questions: Handcrafting the standardized questionnaire.* Beverly Hills, CA: Sage Publications, 1986.
36. Deyo RA, Patrick D. Barriers to the use of health status measures in clinical investigation, patient care, and policy research. *Med Care* 27 (Supp): 5254–5268, 1989.
37. Deyo RA, Inui TS. Toward clinical applications of health status measures: Sensitivity of scales to clinically important changes. *Hlth Serv Res* 19:276–289, 1984.
38. Deyo RA, Centor RM. Assessing the responsiveness of functional scales to clinical changes: An analogy to diagnostic test performance. *J Chron Dis* 39:897–906.
39. Miller GA. The magical number seven, plus or minus two: Some limits on our capacity for processing information. *Psychol Rev* 63:81–97, 1959.
40. Osgood C, Suci G, Tannenbaum P. *The measurement of meaning.* Urbana: University of Illinois Press, 1957.
41. Brook RH, Ware JE, Rogers WH, et al. Does free care improve adults' health? *N Engl J Med* 309:1426–1434, 1983.
42. Stewart AL, Greenfield S, Hays RD, et al. Functional status and well being of patients with chronic conditions: Results from the Medical Outcomes Study. *JAMA* 262:907–913, 1989.
43. Nelson EC, Landgraf JM, Hays RD, et al. The COOP function charts: A set of single item health status measures for use in clinical practice. In Stewart AL, Ware JE (eds). *Measuring Functional and Well-Being: The Medical Outcome Study Approach* (Manuscript submitted for publication).
44. Nelson EC, Wasson J, Kirk J, et al. Assessment of function in routine clinical

practice: Description of the COOP chart method and preliminary findings. *J Chron Dis* 40 (Suppl): 55S–63S, 1987.

45. Berry S. Methods of data collection and ensuring respondent cooperation. In Stewart AL, Ware JE (eds) *Measuring Functional Status and Well-Being: The Medical Outcomes Study Approach* (Manuscript submitted for publication).

46. Jette AM, Davies AR, Cleary PD, et al. The Functional Status Questionnaire: Reliability and validity when used in primary care. *J Gen Int Med* 1:143–1986.

47. Stewart AL, Hays RD, Ware JE, Bindman A. The MOS Short-Form General Health Survey: Reliability and validity in a patient and a disadvantaged population. In Stewart AL, Ware JE (eds). *Measuring Functional Status and Well-Being: The Medical Outcomes Study Approach* (Manuscript submitted for publication).

48. Tarlov AR. Shattuck Lecture—the increasing supply of physicians, the changing structure of the health services system, and the future practice of medicine. *N Engl J Med* 308:1235, 1983.

49. Ellwood P. Shattuck lecture—outcomes management—a technology of patient experience. *N Engl J Med* 318: 1549–1556, 1988.

50. American College of Physicians Health and Public Policy Committee. Comprehensive functional assessment for elderly patients. *Ann Int Med* 109:70–72, 1988.

51. Rubenstein LV, Calkins DR, Young RT, Fink A, Delbanco TL, Brook RH. Improving patient functional status: Can questionnaires help? *Clin Res* 34:835A, 1986.

52. Calkins DR, Rubenstein LV, Cleary PD, Jette AM, Brook RH, Delbanco TL. The functional status questionnaire: A controlled trial in a hospital based practice. *Clin Res* 34:359A, 1986.

53. Kazis LE, Meenan RF, Anderson JJ, Swift MA. The clinical utility of health status information in rheumatoid arthritis patients: A controlled trial. *Arth Rheum* 30 (4) (Suppl): S12, 1987.

2
The Development of a New Measuring Instrument

T.B. ROGERS

Introduction

The goal of this chapter is to examine the measurement of patient functioning as an assessment problem. This will be accomplished by comparing this domain with a number of others, and outlining some of the features of patient functioning that mark it as unique. Such a comparative approach will render visible some of the basic issues, that confront any attempt to proceed with the measurement of patient functioning. So, too, does comparison with developments in other domains point to several methodological approaches that might be appropriate should WONCA decide to begin the process of measure development.

The domain of patient functioning is very complex and poses a number of special measurement problems. This complexity is exacerbated by a set of constraints imposed by the mandate of WONCA, yielding what I believe to be a measurement challenge of great proportions. Yet, there is remarkable similarity with domains such as personality assessment, teaching evaluation, and program evaluation. A comparison with these domains is quite instructive and promises a number of benefits, including: (i) a culling of the expertise developed in these fields, which may be useful in the present context; (ii) the identification of the unique characteristics of the domain, which may signal the need for unusual development strategies; and (iii) the articulation of a number of questions that should be asked in the interest of avoiding some of the difficulties that are encountered in other domains.

The Measurement of Patient Functioning as a Rank Reduction Exercise

At root, the fundamental challenge in the measurement of patient functioning is to synthesize—or to boil down—an incredibly large observational base related to perceptions about health into a workable set of dimensions. In a sense, the task is to develop an effective shorthand that will capture the basic characteristics of patient well-being. This shorthand must be short (i.e., more efficient than asking all possible questions about health) but also representative (i.e., containing as much relevant information as possible). Should such an instrument become available it will be possible to (i) enhance the quality of the patient–physician encounter by providing a systematic information base; (ii) make ipsative (i.e., within patient) analyses of disease progression; (iii) compare various treatment approaches; and (iv) permit the comparison of medical experience between countries.

The challenge of patient functioning assessment can be characterized as a fundamental "rank reduction" exercise in which the goal is to crystallize the immensely complex domain of patient functioning into a number of workable dimensions. The term *rank reduction* comes from multivariate statistics (e.g., factor analysis) in which the goal is to reduce an informational set to the smallest number of essential dimensions (or factors) representing as much of the information as is reasonable. This process of moving from a large informational set to a smaller number of underlying dimensions is called rank reduction which is a relatively apt description of the problem confronting the measurement of patient functioning.

In patient functioning, the initial informational base to be reduced is incredibly complex. It involves a large number of possible judgments about health status, ranging from relatively simple physical attributes to immensely complex concerns of social functioning. There is a wide range of potential information that could, conceivably, be included in the domain, which indicates the need for considerable reduction in the eventual instrument.

The task before WONCA is even more complex because of the almost infinite number of contexts from which data are to be gathered and for which the selected synthesis will have to be relevant. Here I mention a few: (i) the desire for the instrument to be effective across almost all disease categories, (ii) the need for multilanguage forms, and (iii) the hope that the instrument will be useful across various cultures and world views. In other words, the domain to be reduced is itself complex, but it is also represented across a number of different contexts. The observational base is, almost literally, infinite— representing an impressive amount of information from a multitude of different contexts. Yet a functional instrument will have to terminate in a functional instrument which contains a workable number of dimensions capturing the essence of patient functioning. Clearly, this is a rank reduction exercise of great proportions.

But added to this is yet another series of constraints that relate to the pragmatic utility of the obtained set of dimensions. For example, the obtained dimensional set should (i) contain as few dimensions as possible to permit rapid assessment; (ii) be compatible with other aspects of WONCA standards; (iii) demonstrate congeniality with the usual patterns of thought of family physicians; (iv) be sufficiently sensitive across the range of possible health (positive through negative) to permit the monitoring of interventions; and (v) demonstrate adequate levels of validity and reliability. These constraints will have to guide the rank reduction exercise. They impose severe limitations on the nature of any efforts to reduce the rank of the observational base. Clearly, this is a considerable challenge.

Bandwidth–Fidelity Dilemma

To reduce such a large and rich observational base into a minimal set of dimensions, under the constraints imposed, automatically locks researchers into one horn of what is called the bandwidth–fidelity dilemma. Bandwidth, in information theory terms,* refers to the range of observations a dimension is intended to summarize. In the case of patient functioning, the bandwidth is exceedingly wide—perhaps as wide as any domain I have encountered.

Unfortunately, in any system, bandwidth is purchased at the expense of fidelity. The more information you attempt to fit onto a 12-in. LP recording, the greater the loss of fidelity. The slower you run a recording tape, the more information you store per unit length, but the poorer the sound quality.†

To encapsulate a wide range of variables such as patient functioning to maintain a narrow bandwidth inevitably will cause a loss of fidelity. That is, the researchers will—by definition—be forced to sacrifice a degree of measurement fidelity in this area if they wish to retain the bandwidth demanded of the measurement context. Here is a real problem that will have to be met head on if we want to develop an acceptable measure of patient functioning.

Perhaps one of the most problematic aspects of this is that the psychometric ideal is a test with high fidelity and narrow bandwidth. In previous psychometric applications, the "good" test attempts to answer just one, very constricted question with great accuracy. For example, a college aptitude test tries to assess one characteristic, ability, very accurately—or with great fidelity. To achieve this it includes numerous redundant items to increase homogeneity and reliability.

Patient functioning, both by virtue of the domain and the constraints being applied to it, is wide bandwidth—hence, low fidelity. This immediately signals a potential conflict between the psychometric ideal and the needs of the patient functioning domain. To the extent that measures of patient functioning are

---

*For the original formulation of the bandwidth–fidelity dilemma, see Shannon and Weaver (1). Adaptations of the notion to the assessment field can be found in Cronbach and Gleser (2) and Cronbach (3).

†I suppose this metaphor with communication systems should be moderated by such recent technological advances as compact disks and information bubbles, wherein physical space does not appear to limit information storage capability. However, even in the miniaturized and digitized world of laser technology, the number of bits required to store information with high fidelity is greater than the number required for less faithful reproduction. All that has really changed is the absolute size of the storage medium—not the trading relationship between bandwidth and fidelity.

guided by classical psychometric criteria such as reliability and validity* there will be a continual and inevitable conflict with the classical psychometric perspective. For example, a psychometric evaluation of the wide bandwidth COOP five-point pain scale (5) compared to a narrow bandwidth scale for the measurement of the same characteristic would, inevitably favor the latter because it more clearly conforms to classical psychometric criteria. In part, this is because the experience of pain is multidimensional [e.g., Bonica and Ventafridda (6)], with aspects such as intensity and periodicity being confounded in the wide bandwidth measure. Research has also indicated that the experience of pain is deeply affected by contextual variables [e.g., Gracely and Dubner (7)], which indicates that a simple scale may prove to be very difficult to justify. Also, the lack of replicated items in the wide bandwidth scale makes the evaluation of traditionally valued properties such as reliability almost impossible.

The wide bandwidth characteristic of patient functioning measurement, therefore, renders it somewhat unique in relation to standard psychometric examples. It is worth keeping this observation in mind as we explore some of the other aspects of the domain and attempt to formulate a viable research strategy.

The Variety of Dimensional Structures Already Articulated

A number of efforts to reduce the wide bandwidth domain of patient functioning to a set of workable dimensions has been presented in the literature. Even a preliminary reading of these efforts reveals considerable variability in both the number and nature of the proposed dimensions. Table 2.1 shows a somewhat representative list of some of the dimensional structures suggested in the literature. The number and the nature of the dimensions appear to vary, even within this very restricted subsample of the available research. At the low end of the scale is the idea that one question is adequate: "How do you feel today" with four possible answers: excellent, good, fair, or poor. The initials of these response alternatives comprise the acronym EGFP. At the high end of the scale is West's work (14) which suggests 32 dimensions to underlie patient functioning.

Table 2.1, rather than being an overview of the field, serves to demonstrate the extent of variation that has been proposed to date. My expectation, based upon the experience of other domains such as teaching evaluation and personality, is that further research will only add to this variation—not reduce

---

*There are numerous instances of calls for reliability and validity in the patient functioning domain and related domains. For an example, see Schipper and Levitt (4).

TABLE 2.1. A sampler of dimensional spaces thought to underlie patient functioning.

Number of dimensions	Dimensions	References
One	Overall rating (EGFP)	8, 9
Four	Physical/occupational function; psychological state; sociability; somatic discomfort	4
Five	Genetic; biochemical; functional condition; mental condition; health potential	8
Five	Disease-specific indicators; physical functioning; emotional functioning; social functioning; general health perceptions	10, 11
Six	Basic activities of daily living; intermediate activities of daily life; mental health; work performance; social activity; quality of interaction	FSQ: 12
Nine	Physical condition; emotional condition; daily work; social activities; pain; change in condition; overall condition; social support; quality of life	COOP: 5
Fourteen	Social interaction; ambulation or locomotion activity; sleep and rest activity; taking nutrition; usual daily work; household management; mobility and confinement; movement of body; communication activity; leisure pastimes and recreation; intellectual functioning; interaction with family members; emotions, feelings, and sensations; personal hygiene	SIP: 13

it. Yet the task of WONCA is to try and find a consensus within this field that is characterized by an already high, and probably increasing variability in the proposed dimensional structure of the domain being addressed. The desire to have a single scale (or set of dimensions) that characterize patient functioning can be to be seen as fundamentally in conflict with the natural progression of research in a field. The natural progression of research in rank reduction contexts is inevitably toward increased variability—not consensus.* Again, as noted with the bandwidth issue, there are aspects of WONCA's mandate that are at variance with the traditional practice in and history of the measurement field. This signals a need for considerable care when the criteria that will be evoked to evaluate the usefulness of various approaches to the measurement of patient functioning are decided upon.

It should be noted here that the nature of the dimensional structure underlying an assessment battery is the fundamental focus of construct validity. Very broadly an instrument has construct validity in proportion to the extent to which it is integrated within a clear theoretical framework. In the

---

*A reading of the chronological development of rank reduction domains such as intelligence and personality assessment reveals a consistent trend toward a finer and finer level of analysis (i.e., more and varied underlying dimensions) as research progresses. For example, see chapters 9 and 17 in Anastasi (15).

original formulation of this important form of validity,* the idea of a nomological network was introduced. The nomological network was thought to communicate the idea that tests *must* be related to specific theoretical constructs if they were to be acceptable. In the case of multiscale batteries, the underlying dimensional structure is the equivalent of the constructs demanding validation. Thus, the postulated dimensional structure is an integral part of construct validity, with the task of the test developer being to present data that support the constructs as hypothesized. An important question, then, becomes the manner in which the dimensional structure has been subjected to empirical scrutiny.

Approaches of Rank Reduction

In reading the literature upon which Table 2.1 is based, it appears that the manner in which the rank of the domain had been reduced received little, if any, consideration. I was unable to find any clear explanation of why a specific set of dimensions had been selected. There was a paucity of explanations concerning the number of dimensions selected as well. One study (13) mentioned the use of "standard sorting procedures," which is quite uninformative. Most of the researchers did not mention the manner in which they arrived at their set of dimensions.† This, of course, raises questions about the construct validity of the instruments.

The most likely manner in which these dimensional structures were formulated involves the use of what might best be described as purely rational processes. Various researchers, using their intuitive understanding of the domain, selected a set of dimensions that appeared to cover the domain as they saw it. Pragmatic concerns, such as requests by potential users, may have entered into the choice as well. Of particular note here is the apparent failure to subject these dimensional structures to empirical scrutiny.

This purely rational approach has some advantages. For example, reducing the rank of the domain in this manner probably enhances the congeniality of the instrument to physicians' typical patterns of thought. If the same fundamental rational processes underlie the scale as underlie physicians' patterns of thought in their day-to-day practices, the obtained instrument will, more than likely, be compatible. This is an important aspect of any scale development, as the wisdom of practitioners is an invaluable and essential

---

*There is some curious history here. Construct validity was introduced very briefly in the American Psychological Association Technical Recommendations for Tests in 1954 (16), defining it an essential characteristic of tests. It was not until a year later that Cronbach and Meehl (17) published a full-blown definition of the idea. Since then, construct validity has grown to be considered *the validity of validities* [see Messick, (18)].
†The same observation holds true for the presentations made during this symposium.

resource in any development exercise. In addition, the rational approach is relatively inexpensive.

But these strengths are very seriously outweighed by the weaknesses inherent in this kind of strictly rational, rank reduction procedure. Here I draw, in metaphorical fashion, from the domain of personality assessment, which has been grappling with this fundamental problem for over 70 years. This is not to suggest that the domain of personality assessment is without its troubles,* but rather it demonstrates the nature of the kinds of criticisms that can evolve from a strictly rational approach to rank reduction.

Drawing from the personality assessment literature, one can see that a most serious weakness of a strictly rational approach to rank reduction is that one cannot help but impart serious biases and unarticulated assumptions onto the domain. If there is no empirical check on the generality, clarity, and potential utility of the dimensional structure, it is entirely possible that the obtained structure will be of limited utility—except to its authors. Advocacy for a measurement instrument becomes an advocacy for one person's view of the domain, and the probability of achieving consensus is minimal.

In the WONCA case, this is particularly problematic, as the goal is to provide a device that will be accepted across a wide range of contexts, and unarticulated assumptions and biases in the manner of rank reduction will be a real problem. Physicians would, rightly, be able to reject the instrument if it didn't agree with their view of the manner in which the domain should be reduced. Only empirical research into the generality and robustness of the structure will prevent this from happening. Such research would provide a necessary level of rhetoric and persuasive communication about the utility of the obtained instrument.

The use of a strictly rational approach to rank reduction also denies some important aspects of the history of assessment. For example, during World War I, J.S. Woodworth attempted to develop a measure that would predict which soldiers would suffer from shell shock or war neurosis. He employed a strictly rational approach in which he identified symptom-like statements that he felt would be good early indicators of shell shock. These were translated into statements to which soldiers could respond "yes" or "no." The prediction about shell shock was derived by counting the number of symptoms the respondent endorsed, with higher numbers suggesting a greater propensity to shell shock. The eventual scale was marginally successful—and Woodworth's methodology prompted major growth in instruments of this type.

However, when subjected to empirical scrutiny, inevitably, instruments such as Woodworth's and the work flowing from this tradition over the next decades were open to attack. Here are some quotations to describe the period:

Investigation fairly consistently confirms the low worth of the most widely publicized instruments (20) (p. 270).

---

*In fact, this area of assessment is in continual difficulty. For example see Mischel (19).

There are some 500 personality tests, most of which are of little or no value as measurement devices. A few, probably not more than a dozen, could be recommended for experimental use in a testing program (21) (p. 9).

Associated with this approach, which involves assembling scales upon an a priori basis, is the assumption that the psychologist building the test has sufficient insights into the dynamics of verbal behavior and its relation to the inner core of personality that he is able to predict beforehand what certain sorts of people will say about themselves. The fallacious character of this procedure has been shown by empirical results.... It is suggested that the relative uselessness of most structured personality tests is due more to a priori item construction than to the fact of their being structured (22) (p. 297).

I submit that continuing to steer the purely rational or a priori course in the domain of patient functioning will lead to a recycling of this level of criticism and blunt the utility and acceptability of any instrument that WONCA decides to sanction.

In the domain of personality assessment, the first response to these criticisms involved a major swing of the pendulum, wherein virtually all rational or a priori considerations were abandoned in favor of strictly empirical strategies. Rather than thinking about how to organize a domain, researchers argued that the dimensional structure and issues such as item selection ought to be determined solely by recourse to empirical data.

Perhaps the best-known example of this radically empirical approach is the Minnesota Multiphasic Personality Inventory (MMPI) (23). Here, a set of statements reflecting certain symptoms, which were answerable as "true" or "false", was administered to a diagnostic group (e.g., depressive patients) as well as to a group of normal subjects. Statistical tests were performed to determine if any of the items were answered differently by the two groups. Items showing meaningful inter-group differences were then assembled to form a scale intended to predict membership in the diagnostic category. For our purposes, it is important to note that there is no recourse to rational considerations whatsoever in this method—rather, the data make all of the decisions about which item goes where.

Although the MMPI emerged as a significant test a number of problems unfolded as the inventory was subjected to intensive evaluation. It was found that the dimensional structure derived from empirical methodologies bore little if any resemblance to the domain it was supposed to represent.* Subsequent developments, particularly the introduction of construct validity, have indicated, rather clearly, that a strictly empirical approach is not the solution either. Some middle ground appears to be needed.

---

*For example, when the dimensional structure of the MMPI was appraised it was found that the 10 basic clinical scales could be reduced to *two* dimensions! Although the nature of these dimensions has been hotly debated [e.g., see Jackson and Messick (24) and Block (25)], the failure to evaluate critically the underlying dimensional structure created major difficulties.

Another purportedly a-rational approach to measurement has also emerged. This involves the use of the multivariate rank reduction methodology known as *factor analysis*. Here, a complex domain is subjected to mathematical rank reduction procedures to provide estimates of the number and nature of underlying dimensions in the domain.* In personality assessment, the best-known application of this methodology is Cattell's Sixteen Personality Factor Questionnaire (16PF) (27), the name of which signals the number of dimensions determined to underlie personality.[†] In large measure it was thought that the analytic procedure could make decisions about the nature of an underlying dimensional structure—again suggesting a relatively a-rational procedure.

But factor analytic methodology is not a panacea either. There are a number of decisions that the factor analyst has to make, which in fact, have a considerable impact upon the nature of the factor structure obtained. For example, the criteria for deciding how many factors warrant being included in an obtained solution are somewhat "loose" [e.g., see Cliff (29)]. The manner in which the final solution is presented (e.g., the rotation of axes in multidimensional space) also has a significant impact upon the nature of the obtained dimensions [e.g., see Guertin and Bailey (30)]. Also, factor structure can readily be manipulated by the set of items going into the analysis in the first place. For example, in measuring aggression, it is possible to gain one factor structure by including only items dealing with verbal manifestations of the trait, whereas a completely different structure can be obtained by sampling other possible manifestations. Clearly, then, the factor analytic method, although it has a place in the development of a dimensional structure, ought not to be considered the only possible method that can be used.

Based upon previous generations of research, the contemporary view espouses an approach that both embraces and combines all three approaches (i.e., rational, empirical, and mathematical/factor analytic) to rank reduction and test development. Such an eclectic approach is thought to be the optimal strategy at this point. Either one of the three approaches considered alone has significant weaknesses, but when they are combined, they give the test developer a very powerful toolbox.

Perhaps the most cited example of an instrument deriving from this combined orientation is the Personality Research Form (PRF) (31). Because it uses an impressive sequential method that incorporates construct validity concerns from the onset, the PRF represents a very strong application of a combined rational and empirical strategy. Once a construct is clarified and defined, items are rationally developed to reflect it. A rigorous selection process follows when items are selected to maximize construct validity viewed

---

*Cohen et al. (26) have given a highly readable description of this method (pp. 621–628).

[†]As with patient functioning, the variety of dimensional structures in the literature is impressive, varying from 1 or 2 [e.g., Eysenck (28)] through 16 [Cattell et al. (27)].

from a diverse number of perspectives. The scales obtained from this approach have demonstrated impressive degrees of reliability and validity, which suggest that the gains of this painstaking development procedure are well worth its costs.*

A Plan

The past 70 years of experience in the personality assessment domain can be translated into a research plan that warrants consideration by WONCA. In this plan, it is suggested that the primary focus should be upon the dimensional structure thought to underlie patient functioning. Rather than ignore this critical aspect of the development process, I believe WONCA should take the lead in articulating the need for clarification of the structure, and perhaps take an active hand in conducting some of the research. I believe that the technological challenge of developing instruments to reflect the dimensions in different language and cultural contexts is minimal, with adaptations of methods such as those pioneered by Jackson being available. The real challenge lies in the development of a generalizable and empirically grounded dimensional structure that is acceptable for use at WONCA sites.

The failure to present a defensible dimensional structure will, inevitably, result in an instrument of questionable utility and acceptability. In a very real sense, the best approach for WONCA involves a research program to decipher an appropriate dimensional structure to represent the domain of patient functioning. The creation of measures to reflect this structure is a (relatively) simple technological problem—but without a consensual and empirically developed structure, the project has little hope of success.

In very broad brush strokes, the proposed plan is as follows:

(a) An exceedingly careful scrutiny of the dimensional sets thought to underlie patient functioning to obtain clarity of definition and usefulness of obtained scores should be performed. Elimination of personal biases and the creation of publicly documentable arguments tracing the reasons for the selections will have to be generated. This should culminate in a proposed structure that fits the pragmatic needs of the domain, while maximizing the potential for cross-contextual applicability.

(b) Conducting empirical studies to explore the manner in which this structure remains intact across some of the contexts in which the instrument will eventually be used. Studies exploring the manner in which the structure

---

*A detailed presentation of this methodology is beyond the scope of this chapter. Jackson has discussed the method in detail in two articles (32, 33) and a book (31). Any adaptation of this approach to patient functioning will have to deal with issues of wide bandwidth and dimensional structure presented earlier, meaning that a considerable revision of Jackson's methods may be necessary.

holds up in different linguistic environments will be particularly important here, if the eventual instrument is to be useful.

(c) The use of contemporary and eclectic methodologies to develop robust and efficient measures of the dimensions. Again, publicly documentable arguments relating the scales to the dimensions will be required.

(d) Execute a series of studies to demonstrate the utility and sensitivity to change of the obtained scales.

This plan will culminate in a set of scales that will have the maximal potential of fulfilling WONCA's mandate.

I would like to underscore the importance of the first two steps in this plan. Although it may seem intuitively obvious to the reader that a specific manner of dimensionalizing patient functioning is "right," this does not mean that it does so to someone else. Even the most seemingly simple distinction between physical and mental functioning (as proposed in most of the structures presented in Table 2.1) may not be intuitively obvious in a culture that does not share our Western notion of the Cartesian dualism between mind and body.* To be sure, a scale assessing daily work will not be intuitively obvious in a culture that does not divide its time between work and play the way we do [for a good example of this, see Toelken (34)]. Finally, scales relating to social support will have radically different meanings and significances in cultures that have different approaches to social support.† These several points underscore the need to be very careful in the determination of the structure thought to underlie patient functioning if the goal is to develop a general instrument.

The plan presented above has a number of advantages that warrant mention. These include (i) the constructs underlying the scales will be fully articulated and consensually acceptable; (ii) the instruments will incorporate state-of-the-art development technologies; (iii) the dimensional structure underlying the scales will be clearly congenial to the major application of the instrument in physicians' offices; and (iv) the construct validity of the scales will be maximized. I believe that the proposed plan is a viable strategy for WONCA to accept in the interests of developing a truly useful and meaningful measure of patient functioning.

Considerations to Guide the Research Plan

As indicated above, assessment of patient functioning presents a number of unique problems to the test developer. In what follows, the manner in which these unique characteristics have an impact on the development process will

---

*For example, Buddhist traditionalists are not at all comfortable with the manner in which we separate the mind from the body.

†Perhaps the most simple example here is to consider the social support differences between American and Japanese cultures.

be discussed. These issues call into question some aspects of the traditional evaluative criteria for tests (e.g., reliability) and also underscore the need for a substantial amount of research in certain areas of the development process.

Reliability. It has always been touted as a "motherhood" issue in measurement. Starting in 1904 with Spearman's historical proposal (35) regarding "correction for attenuation,"* the notion of reliability has occupied a central place in assessment. In very rough terms, reliability is considered to be the error-free component of a test score. In the usual application, this is estimated by giving a test twice, separated by a suitable time interval. The size of the correlation between the results of the two testings is thought to be an index of the test's reliability. The ultimate by this criterion would be a test for which all respondents receive exactly the same score upon both administrations (i.e., the reliability would be 1.00 in this case).

But in the patient functioning context, this is not the definition of the "ultimate" test. The goal is *not* a test in which everyone obtains the same score upon successive administrations—rather, what is needed is a test that will be sensitive to therapeutic intervention. A perfectly reliable test would be useless in the patient functioning domain. It appears that the classical notion of reliability is not salient in the present measurement situation.[†]

In classical psychometrics, the usual response to this problem is to suggest that there is another kind of reliability that should be considered. This second kind of reliability requires only one administration of a test. For example, you could develop two half scores—one based upon the odd-numbered items, and one upon the even-numbered items—or some such division. A high corelation between these would indicate that the test was reliable within one administration. Sophisticated methods of calculating these correlations have evolved (36, 37) and have become known as measures of homogeneity or internal consistency.

However, in the domain of patient functioning, there is a problem with measures of internal consistency. Practical constraints upon the testing experience—for example, making it short—almost rule out any possibility of replicating observations. It is highly unlikely that it will be possible to include, say, a 20-item scale in the assessment of one component of patient functioning because of time constraints. However, a measure of internal consistency requires replicated items to permit the calculation of the reliability coefficient. To the extent that the desire is for single-item scales [e.g., Nelson et al. (5)], it will not be possible to calculate measures of internal consistency.

---

*The correction for attenuation was the forerunner of the contemporary idea of test–retest reliability and was formulated by Spearman in 1904 (35).

†Stated a bit more forcefully, it would appear that the domain of patient functioning needs *unreliable* tests–ones that change on successive administrations. A demonstration of high test–retest reliabilities for a scale in this context would not be useful information.

In a very real sense, the measurement of patient functioning presents a unique and fundamental challenge to the classical notion of reliability. To adopt the criteria of reliability unthinkingly will result in having to fit the scale, in a rather Procrustean manner, into an inappropriate set of criteria. As with the notion of patient functioning being a wide band–low fidelity domain, so too are the classical ideas of reliability problematic.

Validity. As indicated above, the focus of a test of patient functioning should be construct validity—an evaluation of the degree to which the instrument is integrated into a viable theoretical account of the patient functioning domain. The research plan presented above has been formulated with exactly this criterion in mind.

Other classical forms of validity are of marginal importance. Predictive validity is not a basic concern, except to the extent the test predicts how patients feel about their health at a given time. This is easily assessed by demonstrating relationships with global measures of functioning, such as the EGFP approach outlined above. Content validity is not overly relevant because of the extent of the rank reduction. The scale will be very abstract, and if the obtained dimensional structures "covers the waterfront," then content validity will have been established.

It would seem clear, then, that the research program should be guided by concerns about construct validity. Without doubt, the best way of ensuring that construct validity is achieved is to follow, very carefully, the proposals in the first two steps of the research plan presented earlier.

Validity Generalization. Another issue that will have to be considered relates to the generalizability of reliability and validity information. Considerable research has indicated that validity information gathered in one situation (e.g., a research context) is not necessarily valid when the test is used in another situation (e.g., a clinical setting). For example, Bennett et al. (38) found considerable variability in the sizes of validity coefficients for standardized aptitude tests as a function of the courses that were being used as criteria and the settings in which the data were collected. This situation-specificity has created a degree of pessimism regarding the generalizability of validity information across situations [see (39) for a review].

This is particularly problematic for the patient functioning area, since the goal is to develop an instrument that will be useful across a wide range of possible contexts (see above). For example, there is a clear desire for the eventual instrument to serve both clinical and research purposes. Some recent research has indicated, rather clearly, that validity information from a research setting does not generalize to clinical application (40). *This means that any instrument put forward by WONCA will have to demonstrate validity for the situation in which it is recommended for use.* This is, clearly, a very significant burden of research, given the wide diversity of situations under which and contexts in which the eventual instrument is to be used.

These discussions of reliability, validity, and generalizability indicate three of the fundamental areas of concern that will have to be addressed by WONCA in order to develop a viable instrument for the measurement of patient functioning. The wide bandwidth characteristics of the domain and the problems this offers classical psychometric criteria make this a very challenging measurement domain.

The appraisals of reliability, validity, and generalizability are not intended to suggest that there is no need for rigorous and systematic evaluation research for an instrument of patient functioning. On the contrary, because of the wide bandwidth aspect of the domain there is an even greater need for rigorous scientific and empirical work. Failure to do this work will eventuate in the failure of the entire enterprise, since the hard-headed work is an integral part of the rhetoric that will accompany any eventual instrument.

However, careful scrutiny ought to be given to the criteria that guide the research program. Blind, unthinking acceptance of criteria developed in narrow bandwidth contexts, which characterize almost all successful measurement applications, is a mistake. The research should be guided by an intelligent and informed set of assumptions that work with, rather than against, the eventual emergence of a useful and defensible instrument to measure patient functioning.

Acknowledgment. Preparation of this manuscript was aided by a grant from the Social Sciences and Humanities Research Council of Canada.

References

1. Shannon C, Weaver W: *The Mathematical Theory of Communication.* Urbana, IL, University of Illinois Press, 1949.
2. Cronbach LJ, Gleser GC: *Psychological Tests and Personnel Decisions.* Urbana, IL, University of Illinois Press, 1965.
3. Cronbach LJ: *Essentials of Psychological Testing, 4th ed.* Cambridge, MA, Harper & Row, 1984.
4. Schipper H, Levitt M: Measuring quality of life: Risks and benefits. *Cancer Treat Reps.* 69(10):1115–1123, 1985.
5. Nelson EC, Landgraf, JM, Hays RD, Wasson JH, Kirk JW: The COOP function charts: A system to measure patient functioning in physicians' offices. Paper presented at symposium on the measurement of patient functioning sponsored by the World Organization of National Colleges, Academies, and Academic Associations of General Practitioners and Family Physicians (WONCA); Calgary, Alberta, October 1988.
6. Bonica JJ, Ventafridda, V (eds): *Advances in Pain Research and Therapy,* Vol 3, New York, Raven Press, 1979.
7. Gracely RH, Dubner R: Reliability and validity of verbal descriptor scales of painfulness. *Pain* 29:175–185, 1987.
8. Bergner M: Measurement of health status. *Med Care* 23(5):696–709, 1985.
9. Ware JE: Monitoring and evaluating health services. *Med Care* 23(5):705–709, 1985.

10. Ware JE: Conceptualizing disease impact and treatment outcomes. Santa Monica, CA: Rand Corporation (unpublished manuscript, 1983).

11. Elford RW, Connis RT, Taylor TR et al: A clinical measure for evaluating patient functioning in diabetes. Draft Manuscript dated May. Also read as a paper at symposium on the measurement of patient functioning sponsored by the World Organization of National Colleges, Academies, and Academic Associations of General Practitioners and Family Physicians (WONCA); Calgary, Alberta, October 1988.

12. Jette AM, Davies AR, Clearly PD, et al: *General Int Med*, 1:143–149, 1986.

13. Gilson BS, Gilson JS, Bergner M, et al: The Sickness Impact Profile: Development of an outcome measure of health care. *Am J Public Health*, 65(12):1304–1310, 1975.

14. West R: Results of the Auckland Health Status Survey. Paper presented at symposium on the measurement of patient functioning sponsored by the World Organization of National Colleges, Academies, and Academic Associations of General Practitioners and Family Physicians (WONCA); Calgary, Alberta, October 1988.

15. Anastasi A: *Psychological Testing, 6th ed.* New York, MacMillan, 1988.

16. American Psychological Association: Technical recommendations for psychological tests and diagnostic techniques. *Psychol Bull* 51:201–238, 1954.

17. Cronbach LJ, Meehl PE: Construct validity in psychological tests. *Psychol Bull* 52:281–302, 1955.

18. Messick S: Constructs and their vicissitudes in educational and psychological measurement. *Psychol Bull* 89:575–588, 1981.

19. Mischel W: *Personality and Assessment.* New York, Wiley, 1968.

20. Watson G: Personality and character measurement. *Rev Educ Res* 8:269–291, 1938.

21. Kornhauser A: Replies of psychologists to a short questionnaire on mental test development, personality, and the Rorschach test. *Educ Psychol Meas* 5:3–15, 1945.

22. Meehl PE: The dynamics of "structured" personality tests. *J Clin Psychol* 1:296–303, 1945.

23. Hathaway SR, McKinley JC: *The Minnesota Multiphasic Personality Inventory*, ed rev. Minneapolis, MN: University of Minnesota Press, 1943.

24. Jackson DN, Messick S: Response styles on the MMPI: Comparison of clinical and normal samples. *J Abnor Social Psychol* 65:285–299, 1962.

25. Block J: *The Challenge of Response Sets.* New York, Appleton-Century Crofts, 1965.

26. Cohen RJ, Montague P, Nathanson LS, Swerdlik ME: *Psychological Testing: An Introduction to Tests and Measurement.* Mountain View, CA: Mayfield, 1988.

27. Cattell RB, Eber HW, Tatsuoka MM: *Handbook for the Sixteen Personality Factor Questionnaire.* Champaign, IL, Institute for Personality and Ability Testing, 1970.

28. Eysenck HJ: *Dimensions of Personality.* London, Kegan Paul, 1947.

29. Cliff N: The eigenvalues-greater-than-one rule and the reliability of components. *Psychol Bull* 103:276–279, 1988.

30. Guertin WH, Bailey JP: *Introduction to Modern Factor Analysis.* Ann Arbor, MI, Edwards Brother, 1970.

31. Jackson DN: *Personality Research Form Manual.* Port Huron, MI: Research Psychologists Press, 1984.

32. Jackson DN: A sequential system for personality scale development, In CD Speilberger (ed): *Current Topics in Clinical and Community Psychology*, Orlando FL: Academic Press, 1970, Vol. 2, pp. 61–96.
33. Jackson DN: The dynamics of structured personality tests. *Psychol Rev* 78:229–248, 1971.
34. Toelken B: *The Dynamics of Folklore*. Boston, MA: Houthton-Mifflin, 1979.
35. Spearman C: The proof and measurement of association between two things. *Am J Psychol* 15, 72–101, 1904.
36. Kuder GF, Richardson MW: The theory of estimation of test reliability. *Psychometrika* 2:151–160, 1937.
37. Cronbach LJ: Coefficient alpha and the internal structure of tests. *Psychometrika* 16:297–334, 1951.
38. Bennett GK, Seashore HG, Wesman A: *Differential Aptitude Tests: Technical Supplement*. Cleveland, OH, Psychological Corporation, 1984.
39. Anastasi A: Evolving concepts of test validation. *Ann Rev Psychol* 37:1–15, 1986.
40. Applegate WB: Uses of assessment instruments in clinical settings. *J Am Geriatri Soc* 35:45–50, 1987.

Part II   Primary Care Considerations

3
The Use of Functional Status Assessment Within the Framework of the International Classification of Primary Care

H. LAMBERTS

Introduction

Health is not an operational concept, function of patients is. Family physicians deal with individuals at those moments in time when they are patients. Function is defined by the Classification Committee of WONCA as the ability of a person to perform in, adapt to, and cope with the given environment, measured both objectively and subjectively over a stated time period. Illness behavior, problem behavior, and health-seeking behavior all refer to specific aspects of function. This is a general concept in family medicine, notwithstanding international differences in the social and cultural context of primary care. It is also accepted that aspects of life, such as spiritual matters, education, socioeconomic conditions, and the political situation, do not directly belong within the frame of reference of family medicine. When the function of patients is disturbed or threatened in the context of a disease or a health problem, physicians and patients can play their respective roles best. As a consequence, it is logical to relate the health problem, the patient's reasons for encounter, and medical interventions to function within the same frame of reference. The International Classification of Primary Care (ICPC) provides a framework to classify reasons for encounter, diagnoses, and interventions. It would be of great advantage if elements of the patient's function could be incorporated in the ICPC.

Defining Elements of Patient–Physician Encounters

The Classification Committee of WONCA has defined essential elements of family medicine with a glossary and with classification systems for diagnoses, reasons for encounter, and diagnostic and therapeutic interventions. (1–4).

Family physicians label the patient's demand for care with a diagnosis and—when useful—they classify it using one of the available classification systems. Labeling a problem as a disease legitimizes the medical interventions that follow. Labeling the patient's demand for care as a nonmedical problem can prohibit entrance into the health care system. The assessment of the utility of medical interventions is based on the desired and the factual changes in the patient's function.

Family physicians use several different diagnostic categories (Figure 3.1). Pathological and pathophysiological diagnoses form the backbone of the medical curriculum and receive the highest professional esteem. Nosological diagnoses lack an indisputable pathological or etiological basis and consequently have an intermediate position, between "real" diseases and the "other" diagnostic categories shown in Figure 3.1, and they depend on medical consensus. Often nosological diagnoses are based on combinations of symptoms and complaints (e.g., neurovegative dysbalance, migraine, irritable bowel syndrome, minimal brain damage, and schizophrenia and many other psychiatric diagnoses). In essence nosological diagnoses are expected to be included in due course in a "higher" category when the etiology and/or pathology have been established. Sometimes, nosological diagnoses are no longer considered a disease (e.g., neurosis, homosexuality) and they are discarded as medical labels.

Symptom diagnoses (e.g., headache, neck pain, fever, tiredness) are important in family practice: often they can be dealt with symptomatologically without the need to establish a "higher" diagnosis.

This applies also when functional complaints, which are related to emotions, are presented to the family physician with the demand for care but cannot be labeled as a pathological entity (e.g., tension headache). Emotions in themselves are not medical entities, and this also applies to most problems of daily life. Most emotions and problems are never presented to a physician with a demand for care and consequently are not considered "diseases." Psychological and social problems that are dealt with during a patient–physician

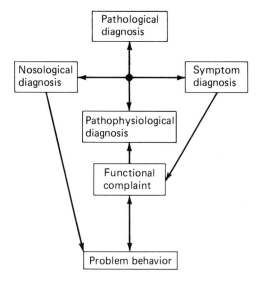

FIGURE 3.1. Diagnostic categories used in family practice.

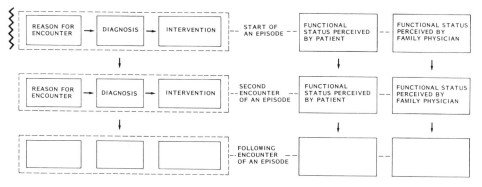

FIGURE 3.2. Relations between encounters in an episode and functional status.

encounter as a problem of life (problem behavior) and not as a disease, however, form an integral part of the daily work in family medicine and have to be included in a classification system for primary care, both as a reason for encounter and as a diagnosis.

It is evident that treatment goals differ considerably among the different diagnostic categories in Figure 3.1. The desired changes in patient function as the consequence of an intervention will vary accordingly.

In addition to different diagnostic categories, differences in clinical judgment between family physicians and specialists, when they treat patients with diseases like diabetes, hypertension, depression, or chronic respiratory disease, have to be taken into account. These differences often are difficult to understand because of the great variability in the course over time ("natural history") of diseases, assessed on the basis of episodes (Figure 3.2) (4). The relations among the patient's reason for encounter or demand for care, the diagnostic interpretation by the physician, and medical interventions and the changes in function that are the consequence form the core of encounters and of episodes. In order to describe and to analyze these relations systematically, a good classification system based on a suitable nomenclature (set of terms) and sufficient terminology (definitions of terms) is needed.

The International Classification of Primary Care

The ICHPPC-2-Defined, IC-Process-PC, and the International Glossary of Primary Care together form the basis for the International Classification of Primary Care (ICPC) (1–4).

The ICPC is a system developed to classify simultaneously three of the four elements of the problem-oriented SOAP registration, as follows:

1. S is for the subjective experience by the patient of his problem, his demand for care, and his reason for encounter as this is clarified by the provider.

CHAPTERS	A-General	B-Blood, blood forming	D-Digestive	F-Eye	H-Ear	K-Circulatory	L-Musculo-skeletal	N-Neurological	P-Psychological	R-Respiratory	S-Skin	T-Metabolic, Endocrine, Nutr	U-Urinary	W-Pregnancy, Childbearing Family Planning	X-Female genital	Y-Male genital	Z-Social
1. Symptoms and complaints																	
2. Diagnostic, screening prevention																	
3. Treatment, procedures, medication																	
4. Test results																	
5. Administrative																	
6. Other																	
7. Diagnoses, disease																	

(left axis label: COMPONENTS)

FIGURE 3.3. Seventeen chapters and their alpha codes and seven components with two digit codes (4).

2. A is for the assessment or diagnostic interpretation of the patient's problem by the provider.
3. P is for the process of care; it represents the diagnostic and therapeutic intervention.
   (The objective findings O cannot be classified with the ICPC.)

The ICPC is a two-axial classification system based on chapters and components. It uses three-digit alphanumeric codes with mnemonic qualities to facilitate its day-to-day use (Figure 3.3).

Seventeen chapters, each with an alpha code, form one axis, while seven components with rubrics bearing a two-digit numeric code form the second axis.

Chapter D (digestive system) illustrates the structure of the classification (Figure 3.4).

The ICPC, as proposed here, is the "gold standard" in the assessment for family medicine of functional status indicators. Feasible, reliable, and valid functional status indicators are directly related to the concepts of the ICPC and consequently can readily be incorporated in the daily work of family physicians. Indicators not directly related to concepts in the ICPC (e.g., happiness, spiritual fulfillment, health perception) are difficult to use in this approach. The question, however, to be answered is whether such indicators describe aspects of function that should be incorporated in the ICPC.

The reverse is true as well. If the ICPC allow us to classify symptoms and complaints, reasons for encounter, diagnoses, and interventions, it can be expected that they all reflect one or more functional status indicators.

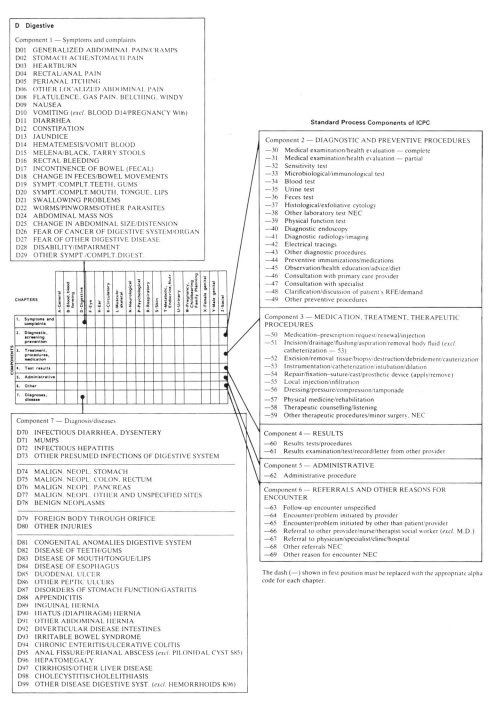

FIGURE 3.4. Chapter D(Digestive) of the ICPC (4). Reprinted with permission from Lamberts H., Wood M. eds. International Classification of Primary Care (ICPC). Oxford, Oxford University Press, 1987.

Essentials of Classification Systems

A classification demands that its user be explicit: What is important, which are the concepts and how are they defined, what are the relations between the concepts, and how can they be measured (5, 6)?

Classification systems are developed to order objects in classes on the basis of their relations. Identification of an object requires assignment to the correct class.

A good classification helps the user (7) to better define the structure of concepts, simplify the relations between concepts, economize on the use of memory, and ease the manipulation and retrieval of data.

A concept is any unit of thought; a term is a word that designates a concept, (8, 9). A classification is the arrangement of concepts into groups or classes, according to established criteria.

It is important to distinguish a nomenclature—the set of terms in the professional jargon—from a classification and a terminology, which include the definition (inclusion criteria) of each term (10) (Figure 3.5). A thesaurus is a storehouse of knowledge that is similar to an exhaustive encyclopedia or a computer file, with a large index and synonyms.

The ICPC follows these principles:

Concepts: symptoms, complaints, reasons for encounter, interventions, diseases, diagnoses
Groups: classes biaxially arranged over components and chapters
Criteria: relevance for family practice; localization before etiology; use of inclusion criteria (terminology); hierarchy in specificity; and one single nomenclature for reason for encounter, diagnoses, and process.

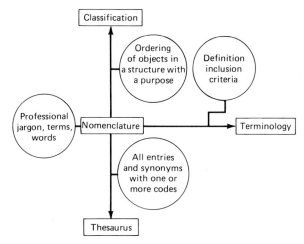

FIGURE 3.5. Differences between a nomenclature, a terminology, a classification, and a thesaurus.

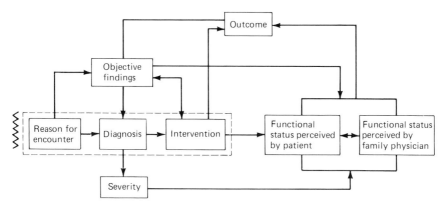

FIGURE 3.6. Indicators in the ICPC framework in which function is distinguished from objective findings, severity of disease, and outcome.

In this framwork, functional status indicators to be used in family practice relate directly with the concepts of the ICPC, they are compatible with the biaxal grouping of classes, and they follow the criteria of relevance and hierarchy in specificity.

To support the incorporation of indicators in the framework of the ICPC, function has to be distinguished from (Figure 3.6) objective findings; severity of disease; and outcome.

For episodes like hypertension, diabetes, and glaucoma, objective findings lead to direct indications for outcome: they do not reflect function directly, but they can help to predict it.

Severity of a disease is also a different clinical concept. Cervical carcinoma or heart failure can have very different consequences for the daily life of a patient according to its severity.

Outcome relates to the formal establishment of the efficacy of an intervention in a randomized, controlled study. Figure 3.6 shows that all the consequences of a disease are related and that the can be distinguished from each other within the structure of encounters and of episodes, as defined by the ICPC.

Practical Consequences

For a good working relation between the ICPC and functional status indicators, five requirements are important:

1. A functional status indicator should reflect validly and reliably a well-defined aspect of function.
2. The content of an indicator must be understood in clinical terms. An aggregated measure, like an index, often does not translate into clinical

concepts and consequently does not allow incorporation in the framework of the ICPC.

3. The patient's self-reported perception of his function must be distinguished from the physician's perception, but the same indicator must be used. Positive and negative discrepancies must also be understood in clinical terms.

4. Indicators are sensitive both to considerable and to relatively small disturbances and changes in function. Many conditions in family practice are of minor importance, but they can temporarily affect the patient's function considerably. In chronic conditions impairment of function can be limited and change over time very slowly.

5. The relation between a therapeutic intervention and the change in function that is its consequence must be understood in clinical terms.

Proposal for the Incorporation of Functional Status Indicators in the Structure of the ICPC

Three elements, as follows, are superimposed on the structure of the ICPC in order to incorporate functional status indicators in it (Figure 3.7): functional status; change over time; and the judge: patient, physician, or both.

The ICPC classifies somatic, psychological, and social problems: it deals with "subjective elements," like the patients symptoms and complaints, and with more "objective" diagnoses.

In this model for each concept in the ICPC, an indicator is possible; it describes the impact of the problem on the function of the patient and the

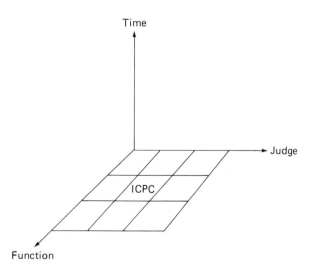

FIGURE 3.7. ICPC as the basis for the use of function indicators.

desired change in function when medical intervention is successful. Limitation of the elements of function that can be incorporated is necessary. Function in the structure of the ICPC as a consequence is limited to symptoms and complaints, health problems, diseases, in different stages of an episode (4).

Rubric -28 in the first component of each chapter of the ICPC is used to designate "disability and impairment" and is the best place to incorporate functional status indicators in the framework of the ICPC. The patient's assessment of his function can be classified in the reason for encounter mode, using rubric -28. The physicians assessment can be classified in the diagnostic or the process mode, also using rubric -28. The practical consequence of this approach can be illustrated with the functional status indicators developed in the COOP project and applied in the Autonomy project. (Nelson, Landgraf, Hays, et al., Chapter 8 and Meyboom-De Jong, Chapter 9, this volume;12).

The COOP charts characterize aspects of function with a five-point scale. (11) (Nelson, Landgraf, Hays, et al., Chapter 8 and Meyboom-De Jong, Chapter 9, this volume; 12). Experiences with the charts, together with the comprehensive use of the ICPC, support the proposal to add a fourth digit to rubric -28 in several ICPC chapters to accommodate, at this moment, five generally accepted, functional status indicators.

The function charts can be coded as:

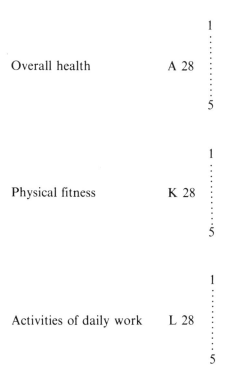

Overall health   A 28

Physical fitness   K 28

Activities of daily work   L 28

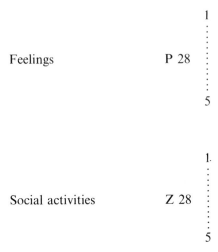

Feelings   P 28

Social activities   Z 28

Pain—also on a five-point scale—can be added as a fourth digit to each ICPC rubric referring to pain, for example,

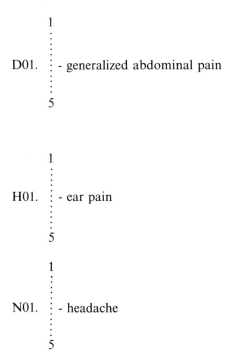

D01.   - generalized abdominal pain

H01.   - ear pain

N01.   - headache

Chapters D(digestive), F(vision), H(hearing), R(respiratory), S(skin), in this proposal, evidently do not have function indicators. New and more specific indicators have to be developed to fit in the structure of the ICPC and they—

hierarchically—can be more specific than the global indicators now included in chapters A, K, L, P, and Z.

The inclusion of an indicator in a certain chapter does not imply that only conditions in the same chapter can be related to this indicator. The ICPC rubrics can be related to all other rubrics in the reason for encounter, the diagnosis, and the process mode.

Change over time is essential to the use of the COOP charts. It is proposed to use

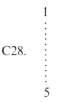

C28.

for this. (C does not refer to an existing ICPC chapter but can easily be incorporated in a patient database coded with the ICPC.)

Conclusion

The ICPC provides a useful framework to support the acceptance and the practical application of functional status indicators in family practice. The available database management systems, based on the ICPC, readily accept additional codes, which is a substantial advantage for registration, coding, data entry, analysis, and interpretation of the data (13).

References

1. Classification Committee of WONCA. *ICHPPC-2-Defined.* (Inclusion Criteria for the Use of the Rubrics of the International Classification of Health Problems in Primary Care.) Oxford, Oxford University Press, 1983.
2. Classification Committee of WONCA. *International Classification of Process in Primary Care (IC-Process-PC).* Oxford, Oxford University Press, 1986.
3. Classification Committee of WONCA. *An International Glossary for Primary Care.* J Fam Pract 13:671–81, 1981.
4. Lamberts H, Wood M, eds. *International Classification of Primary Care (ICPC).* Oxford, Oxford University Press, 1987.
5. Wood M. Family Medicine Classification Systems in evolution. *J Fam Pract* 12:199–200, 1981.
6. Froom J. New directions in standard terminology and classifications for primary care. *Pub Hlth Rets* 99:73–77, 1984.
7. Sokal PR, Classification: Purpose, principles, progress, prospects. *Science* 185:1115–1123, 1974.

8. WHO. *International Nomenclature of Diseases: Guidelines for Selection of Recommended Terms and for Preparation of IND Entries.* Geneva, WHO-Technical Terminology Service, 1987.
9. Nationale Raad voor de Volksgezondheid. *Ontwerp van de WCC. Standaard termen voor classificaties en definities*, 88WCC9. Zoetermeer, 1988.
10. Anonymous. *Principles and Methods of Terminology. Draft International Standard.* Geneva, International Organization for Standardization. ISO/DIS 704, 1985.
11. Nelson E, Conger B, Douglass R, Gephart D, et al. Functional health status levels of primary care patients. *JAMA* 249:3331–3338, 1983.
12. Meyboom-De Jong B. *Bejaarde Patiënten. Een Onderzoek in twaalf huisartspraktijken.* Lelystad, Meditekst, 1989.
13. Lamberts H, Brouwer HJ, Groen ASM, Huisman H. Transition project. Huisarts Wet 30:3–11, 1987.

4
The History of Health Status Assessment from the Point of View of the General Practitioner

B.G. BENTSEN

Introduction

The aim of clinical practice is much more than the diagnosis of disease. The central issue is improvement of patients' functional capacity and well-being. If this cannot be achieved, the minimal goal is to reduce the impact of the disease on a patient's life.

The ultimate aim of medical care should be to reintegrate individuals into the normal productive life of society and not just treat their symptoms or diseases.

For the individual patient, function can be a matter of life or death, and it is the major component of prognosis over time. Health care attempts to improve a patient's level of function or to maintain it if cure is not possible. The rehabilitation process has as its goal restoration placement of function.

A population comprises individuals. Assessment of an individual's functional capacity in relation to treatment, work, rehabilitation, sickness benefits, or pension is also part of defining that population's needs: that is, the planning of health services, insurance systems, social support systems, and community structure or infrastructure.

Assessment of a patient's functional status or health status has been a basis for the generalist's decisions throughout the years. Diagnosis of disease is important from the perspective of function. For subspecialists, it seems that the assessment of organ—or organ system function—has been the central issue.

At present there are no generally accepted instruments for measuring function—or health status. One reason may be the difficulty in defining a frame of reference. What is "normal"? What can be expected? Some persons function exceptionally well throughout their life. Other persons adapt well with limited resources—perhaps even with fewer resources as life goes on.

Is is possible to present standardized instruments for measuring health that can be used in clinical primary practice all over the world and that are suitable for all types of health conditions, stages of illness, and severity of problems? Do we need such instruments?

The History of Health Indicators

Assessment of health has had different goals throughout history. In old Babylon in 1792 BC, we find such an assessment documented in the Laws of Hummurabi (1). The points in Table 4.1 (first column) were related to certain outcomes of health care.

Florence Nightingale, in her "Notes of Hospitals," introduced health indicators in hospitals. She recommended that the outcome of care should be classified as "dead," "relieved," or "unrelieved." This classification is as sophisticated as those in routine use in hospitals today.

Traditionally, measurement of invalidity has been the central issue. Insurance company tables date back to Bismarck in the 1880s and detail compensation to coal miners in Schlessien for loss of income or loss of earning capacity because of accidents in the mines. This is still the rather meaningless basis for compensations and pensions in relation to such accidents.

From the 1940s through the 1950s, several systems for assessment of consequences of disease were developed. The need to determine the physical fitness of recruits in World War II pushed forward the development of a number of assessment scales. Thus, the Pulses Profile was developed from the Canadian Army's "physical Standards and Instructions." The Pulses Profile, published in 1957, measured activities of daily living (ADL) (2). In the NES Survey (1952 through 1955), a similar instrument was used (3). Results from that study are presented below in comment on general practice and the measurement of health.

However, the most effort was made to develop instruments for measuring consequences of single disease processes. We have, for example, one for cardiovascular diseases, one for rheumatoid arthrities, one for multiple sclerosis. This organ system approach reflects a traditional, biomedical, reductive concept. The WHO's "International Classification of Impairments, Disabilities and Handicaps" (4) (1983) follows such a principle. Similarly Feinstein, in his book *Clinimetrics* (5) (1987), states that when he files reports on the many hundreds of different instruments in the literature, he uses organs or organ systems as his filing principle.

The work on health indicators in Europe and North America from the 1960s through the 1970s was important, both from the theoretical and the practical

TABLE 4.1. Utility scale adjusted for socioeconomic ground.

10	Death of freeman/Loss of eye of freeman/Loss of hand of surgeon
5	Death of nobleman/Loss of eye of nobleman/Fracture of limb of freeman/Intestinal obstruction of freeman
3	Fracture of limb of nobleman/Intestinal obstruction of nobleman
2	Death of slave/Loss of eye of salve
0.2	Death of ox

point of view. One objective was to find a general expression for an individual's health status. However, the multitude of instruments that were developed confused these issues.

Recently researchers have tried to assess instruments that measure health and functional status. Of the greatest importance is the work done by McDowell and Newell, which is reported in their *Measuring Health: A Guide to Rating Scales and Questionnaires* (1987) (2). They assessed 50 of the best instruments published on the following indicators: ADL, psychological well-being, social health, quality of life and life satisfaction, pain, and general health measurement. They drew the following conclusions (reprinted with permission):

On Functional Disability and Handicap

Research that compares different scales for measuring physical functional capacity has yet to be done. . . .

On Pyschological Well-Being

The embarrassment of riches: There are many well tested measurements, and it was not easy to set criteria for what should be included. . . serious disadvantages for making piecemeal alterations to the questions in the scale.

On Social Health

How he gets along with other people, how other people react to him, and how he interacts with social institutions and societal mores. [The ever-present] lack of evidence for (the instruments') validity and reliability.

On Quality of Life and Life Statisfaction

Measuring such an abstract and complex a theme as . . . no longer seems presumptuous. [However] quality of life remains more a fashionable idea than a rigorously defined concept in health sciences.

On Pain Measurement

Close attention has been paid to reliability and validity in the development of (pain) measurement methods . . . the link between clinical interests in pain management and the measurement techniques has been closer in this field than in, say, functional disability.

On General Health Measurement

Most recently developed measurement methods. . . (are) a showpiece of current health measurement technology. . . conceptual formulation,. . . reliability and validity, a tendency towards development of alternative versions that are not strictly comparable.

They also represent the major research instruments, as opposed to strictly clinical scales....

The reader will have been struck by the considerable variation in the quality and sophistication of the health measurements presented. This may reflect the relative newness of the field: the development of health indices is a recent endeavor compared with measuring intelligence or public opinion. Certainly, health measurement has benefited from the theoretical and technical advances in test construction already achieved in the social sciences, but the application of this knowledge to health measurements has been uneven. Pain scales seem to have been most successful in exploiting the more sophisticated scaling techniques, while measurements of psychological well-being have devoted the greatest attention to validity testing. Meanwhile, the field of functional disability shows a different picture: the profusion of measurement scales is rivaled only by their lack of technical sophistication. The doubtful quality of many of these scales appears to have fostered the reaction of developing yet more scales, whose superiority is more often assumed then demonstrated. We should now pay closer attention to refining and testing existing instruments than to developing new methods, and when a new method is clearly required its design should be based on a careful analysis of the strengths and weaknesses of previous scales.

On the theme of building on prior experience, we have repeatedly mentioned the desirability of a conceptual definition of the topic being measured. This is intended to stress the role of measurement in scientific discovery: as science ultimately tests theories we must know that theoretical orientation each health index represents. This goal has been quite well achieved in the fields of pain measurement and emotional well-being, and to a certain extent in quality of life measures.

While we may complain about the weakness and lack of coordinated development work in certain areas of health measurement, we must also acknowledge that the universal, perfect index will never exist and that it is impossible to select one set of questions applicable to all diseases and all individuals.

The recently developed Dartmouth COOP instrument (6) is currently being tested. It seems to meet many of the requirements that can be listed in relation to an instrument adaptable for primary care. Of importance in the development of instruments for measuring health has been the focus on reliability and validity. New methods have been developed to make "soft data," like pain or social support, measurable; "the unmeasurable measurable" (2, 5).

The measurement of health have gone through three stages: The question of life or death; disease and the functional capacity of organ systems; and subsequently, a person's functional capacity, or health status.

A Survey From General Practice

Few Studies on the measurement of health or consequences of disease from general/family practice have been published. Bent Guttorm Bentsen's survey from 1952 to 1955 will be cited because it reflects a general practitioner's way of thinking (3). The NES study's goal was to analyze health services and the consequences of disease in a geographically defined population. The preva-

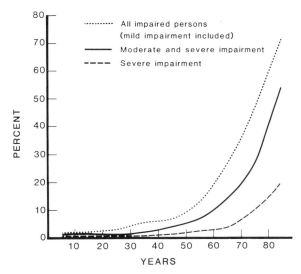

FIGURE 4.1. Point prevalence of permanent impairment. Percentage impaired persons within each 10-year age-group as of 31st December 1955. Activities of daily living and dependency as assessed by physician in a district in Southeast Norway.

lence of impairment as of 31st December 1955 was assessed in a population of 5,646 persons. The population represented an average Norwegian population in relation to many variables. A person was described as "impaired" when he had a "permanently reduced ability to perform the tasks of daily living." The instrument that was developed was nearly identical to the later published PULSES PROFILE (2) and took into account reduced physical and mental functional capacity and dependency. A four-point scale was used: absence of impairment and mild, moderate, and severe impairment. The diseases causing impairment were recorded, as were the economic support and work capacity of the impaired person. Figure 4.1 shows the prevalence of impairment in the population as of 31st December 1955. This could be used as a "good standard" for prevalence of objectively assessed impairment in a population.

The study showed that the most frequent diseases causing impairment were circulatory system diseases (24.5%), mental disorders (17.17%), and musculo-skeletal system diseases (16.4%). An average of 1.5 impairing health problems were recorded per impaired person. Mental disorders had the most serious impact on working capacity (3).

Definitions of Health and Health Status

The World Health Organization's defines *Health* as "a state of complete physical, mental, and social well-being, and not merely the absence of disease or infirmity."

Few people can meet the WHO's definition for health. Either these persons are real deviants (psychotic) or a person who can meet these criteria only at certain moments of life.

WONCA has proposed changing the WHO definition. The word *optimal* is substituted for the word *complete*: *Optimal* physical, mental, and social well-being. That means that health must be assessed relative to the individual's possibilities and living conditions.

Can health be measured? Can well-being the measured? It is possible to do this. However, it is easier to assess their absence: absence of well-being, absence of health, as in the survey described above.

It therefore makes sense that a subcommittee of WONCA has proposed that we should at present focus on intruments measuring absence of health in persons encountered in primary care. Health is not an operational concept, function of patients is. As a consequence family physicians/general practitioners deal with individuals at those moments in time when they are patients.

The accepted definition of *function* is "the ability of a person to perform in, adapt to, and cope with given environment, measured both objectively and subjectively over a stated time period."

Needs for Measuring Functional Status

The slow development of instruments that measure health reflects the general history of modern medicine. Until the 1970s the paradigm of organ-oriented specialties dominated. In the 1980s the "whole person," a holistic concept, has gained momentum.

The WHO definition and the classification of impaired organs or organ systems is difficult to understand. There is no common denominator or variable. The use of the word *impairment* in this way may be helpful in subspecialties, but it is an abstraction in general medical practice.

The function of a person as a whole is more than the sum of functions of separate organ systems. Assessment of the functioning of separate organs or organ systems does not always described how the person actually functions or how well the person performs in his/her daily environment. Separate instruments that assess consequences of disease and the function of organs is not very meaningful to a generalist. Here we need common denominators and variables related to persons. These can only be variables that are independent of organ systems; for example a common denominator for "blindness, hemiplegia, grave mental retardation" could be "difficulties in moving around."

In the introduction it was stressed that the functional status of the patient over time is the central issue in daily practice. Describing a person's health or functional capacity is like describing a die: It can be described by the number of dots on its upturned side: "one" or "six," for example; color; size; or the material it is made of. Similarly a general practitioner needs separate indicators or a profile for health assessment. A summation of these indicators, that is, a health index, is meaningless. The indicators could be physical and mental functioning, dependence, social functioning, working and earning capacity, and use of health services. In addition one would need an assessment of how much the symptom or complaint (e.g., pain or dizziness) hurts or bothers: not at all, somewhat more, or a great deal.

There seems to be little need for an instrument that can be used during every encounter in general practice. However, Nelson et al. (6) have shown that a simple, comprehensive instrument can affect doctor–patient communication. It can give new and important information that can lead to new management activity (6). There is a need to measure the functional status of persons with long-term diseases, elderly persons, and patients with unclear health problems.

In addition to the need for an instrument for use in daily practice, we need instruments that can be used in primary care research. For this purpose instruments can be complex but must be well tested. The type of study will determine which instrument is chosen. For example, a study on the need for a certain community service requires a simpler instrument than is needed to analyze a particular health problem or the effect of its treatment.

Developing a new instrument for use in general practice is not realistic. It is a hopeless challenge. One must choose among those that are well tested and in current use. Very few seem to meet the requirements that will be listed.

Criticisms of instruments were mentioned earlier. The most important are lack of sufficient reliability and validity testing (2). Additional criticisms relate to lack of suitability for a studied population's health problems. Existing instruments are too complex, too time consuming, and too long (i.e., they have too many questions). Those instruments attempting a global health index, instead of a profile, often compare apples and oranges in an overall assessment.

Requirements of Instruments to Assess Functional Status in Daily General/Family Practice

The international academic organization for general practice/family medicine (WONCA) has been cooperating with the WHO to develop primary care classifications and definitions for many years. Regrettably this is no longer being done. It would have been useful for WONCA and WHO to take joint responsibility for the development or choice of instruments to measure health or functional status of primary care patients.

For WONCA this work is the sensible and logical consequence of the WONCA Classification Committee's prior work on classification, criteria, and definitions of terms for primary care. It is useful to relate, if possible, assessment of functional status to ICPC, ICHPPC-2-Defined, IC-Process-PC, and WONCA's glossary of terms (7–9).

The purpose of instruments that measure health or functional status is to provide person-oriented, objective data ordinarily neglected in the clinical encounter. This can permit outcome assessments over time related either to therapies or to the natural history of the disease. This will also make comparisons between practices possible.

Instruments that can be used in daily primary care practice must be:

1. Person-oriented. We aim to draw a profile of indicators that describe a person's functional state. The indicators must be described in clinical terms. The profile could comprise ADL, or a comprehensive bio–psycho–social assessment.
2. Reliable and valid. The test–retest reliability must be high. The instrument must have a high degree of face validity and criterion validity. The instrument must be completely tested in a noninstitutionalized population, and be clinically relevant.
3. Useful. Simplicity is a basic requirement. At most the instrument should contain fewer than 10 questions. However, more complex instruments like GHQ-30 seem to be operational (10). It should also be suitable for all primary care encounters, regardless of the patient's age and sex; for all types of conditions; and for every stage and severity of a problem. The instrument should at minimum cover all important conditions and should be clinically relevant. The instrument should be low-tech, portable, and cheap. It should also be acceptable in the busy daily practice, and easily interpretable scores are required.
4. Sensitive. It should be sensitive for measurements of small changes in health—especially in relation to outcome measures.
5. Internationally acceptable. This requirement is perhaps the most difficult to meet. It implies that the instrument not be limited by culture; thus testing of it all over the world would be required.

The use of an instrument also raises questions about time and administration: When should the assessment take place and who should administer the instrument?

The assessment of function will primarily be limited to a point in time. Repeating the assessment at intervals will make it possible to determine changes. Retrospective consideration of the person's status during the past 6 or 12 months will make it possible to sort out those persons with long-term impairment.

One should expect differences between a person's self-assessment and assessment by a professional. However, the instrument must be acceptable and operational for the three potential administrators: The patient: subjective; the physician: objective; the community: collective norms.

Conclusion

Assessment of health or functional status is important during all encounters between primary care professionals and patients. The medical profession has been slow to develop instruments to measure patient status. There is a need for such intruments in the general/family practitioner's daily practice in other primary care setting, and for research.

Requirements for an instrument to measure health or functional status, applicable in daily practice, seem unattainable. However, methods have been developed and assessed recently. Much may still be lacking in reaching an ideal, internationally acceptable method. What has been done provides a basis for choice for general/family practitioners. A choice between the best tested and relevant instruments must be offered. Promising instruments for general/family practice are still not sufficiently tested, and must be tested further.

To choose methods to measure functional or health status of primary health care patients is no longer impossible. It is possible and we hope, will very soon be a reality.

References

1. Smith GT: *Measuring the Social Benefits of Mediciene.* Off Health Economics, 1983.
2. McDowell I, Newell C: *Measuring Health: A Guide to Rating Scales and Questionnaires.* Oxford/New York, Oxford University Press, 1987.
3. Bentsen BG: Vurdering av invaliditet i en befolkning. *Tidsskr Nor Lægeforen* 30:295–302, 1966. (Assessmet of invalidity in a population). Later published in Bentsen BG: *Illness and General Practice. A Survey of Medical Care in an Inland Population in South-East Norway 1952–1955.* Oslo Bergen Tromsø, University Press, 1986.
4. World Health Organization: International Classifications of Impairements, Disabilities and Handicaps, Geneva, WHO, 1983.
5. Feinstein AR: *Clinimetrics.* New Haven London, Yale University Press, 1987.
6. Nelson EC, et al.: Dartmouth COOP Proposal To Develop and Demonstrate a System To Assess Functional Health status In Physicians Office, Final Report. Hanover, NH, Dartmouth Medical School, 1987.
7. Lamberts H, Wood M: ICPC Working Party: *International Classification of Primary Care.* Oxford University Press, 1987.
8. Classification Committee of WONCA: *ICHPPC-2-Defined* (International Classification of Health Problems in Primary Care). Oxford University Press, 1983.
9. Classification Committee of WONCA in Collaboration with NAPCRG (North American Primary Care Research Group): *IC-Process-PC* (International Classification of Process in Primary Care). Oxford University Press, 1986.
10. Hall J, Hall N, Fisher E, Killer D: Measurement of outcomes of general practice: Comparison of three health status measures. *Fam Pract* 4:117–122, 1987.

5
Disease-Specific Functional Status Assessment

J. FROOM

Introduction

There are several compelling reasons to assess functional status of patients treated by family physicians. Of these reasons, the evaluation of therapeutic interventions as related to clinical outcome, is perhaps the most important. Outcome evaluations are generally made using objective measures, such as reduction in blood pressure, change in selected laboratory values (e.g., serum creatinine and calcium), and crude qualitative patient responses expressed as "less pain" or "feeling better." Yet, even precise laboratory results give an incomplete picture of the clinical situation. A patient taking antihypertensive medication who has achieved normal blood pressure may be incapicitated from the medication's side effects. Chemotherapy can disable the patient in whom there is radiological evidence of tumor regression. Clearly, the current assessment of outcomes of treatment in ambulatory patients is both incomplete and imprecise. Functional status assessment is required in addition to precisely defined clinical end points.

Functional status assessments also provide information that is clinically useful. Evidence of impairment derived from measurements of social isolation, inability to perform tasks of daily living, and dysphoric mood can often be addressed with appropriate therapies and environmental interventions. These self-assessments provide significant prognostic information. For patients over age 75, the risk of death is twofold greater for those who perceive their health as poor as compared with those who perceive their health as good, even when adjusted for disease state and disability (1). Indeed, the needs of this group of patients will be better met by careful assessment of functional status than by precise delineation of their diagnoses. Lastly, during these times of shrinking resources, it is necessary to demonstrate that interventions have benefits commensurate with their costs.

The assessment of functional status is feasible in the ambulatory care setting. The Duke–UNC Health Profile (DUHP) (2), a 63-item instrument, can be self-administered in 10 minutes or less. It has good reliability and validity as supported by strong correlations with the Sickness Impact Profile (3), the

Tennessee Self-concept Scale (4), and the Zung Self-rating Depression Rating (5). A somewhat more complex instrument has been developed by Rae West of New Zealand. It assesses enjoyment of life, vulnerability, daily health disability, and health service utilization. It can be given to ambulatory patients and has been used in a study of terminal cancer patients (6). Perhaps the instruments that can be given most quickly and easily are the Dartmouth COOP function charts (7), developed by E. Nelson and colleagues. In their current form, they consist of nine charts that measure physical condition, emotional condition, daily work, social activities, pain, change in condition, overall condition, social support, and quality of life. Designed with cartoon-assisted descriptions, and a rating scale of 1 to 5, the patient evaluates his/her functional status for each of the nine conditions. Either self-administration or health-provider administration is appropriate.

Although assessment of functional status is both desirable and feasible for the ambulatory patient, it is necessary to address several issues concerning the incorporation of these measures into daily practice. It is also necessary to consider how these assessments will relate to the several classifications devised by the WONCA Classification Committee. These include diagnostic assessments (*ICHPPC-2-Defined*) (8); recording of process (IC-Process-PC) (9); a combined recording of reason for encounter, process, and diagnoses (ICPC) (10); and the "International Glossary for Primary Care" (11). This chapter will address mechanisms to incorporate functional status assessments into daily practice and will include recommendations that relate these assessments to specific diagnoses.

Several Functional Status Assessment Instruments Are Needed

Three types of indices are currently available. The first type measures general health or well-being and is particularly suitable as a screening instrument. The three instruments described above, that is the Duke–UNC-Health Profile, the Dartmouth COOP function charts, and the instrument developed by West are of this type. They are suitable for screening, but it is unclear if they can be used to assess the several components of functional disability associated with specific diseases sufficiently. They could be given to each patient to provide base-line information and periodically to the elderly to assess the combined effect of aging and pathological process. A second type, exemplified by the Arthritis Impact Measurement Scale (12), is intended to measure the physical, social, and emotional well-being of arthritic patients. The third type is designed to assess the consequences of a symptom. An example is the McGill Pain Questionnaire (13), which is designed to follow patients with severe, and chronic pain. A question that requires additional research is the utility and validity of a general well-being instrument, such as the Dartmouth COOP function charts in the assessment of changes in patients with specific chronic diseases (e.g., diabetes or arthritis).

Recording Signs, Symptoms, and Laboratory Results

The major goal of determining the relationship between medical intervention and outcome will not be achieved by functional status assessment alone. It also is necessary to follow the course of diseases under study by carefully recording and measuring signs, symptoms, and laboratory results. We need to quantify these observations, however, to increase the accuracy of outcome assessment. Laboratory results are for the most part reported in units that permit comparisons, but it is also possible and necessary to quantify the duration and severity of a cough or the extent of a skin rash. For example, a burn chart could be used to depict the extent of a skin rash and the severity of a cough can be rated on a Likert scale. It is necessary to choose the signs, symptoms, and laboratory tests that are most suitable to follow the course of specific diseases. These clinical indicators should be linked to the inclusion criteria already developed for the *ICHPPC-2-Defined* (8).

Who Should Receive Functional Assessment?

Information derived from screening all adult patients at an initial encounter with the physician with a general health assessment instrument like the Dartmouth COOP function charts could be useful. Unsuspected disabilities may be uncovered and lead to medical interventions. Other rational uses include periodic screening of geriatric patients and of all patients with chronic illness. The frequency of these assessments will depend upon the type and severity of the disease and is, therefore, a matter of individual clinical judgment. It is unlikely that functional assessments of patients with acute self-limited illnesses, in the absence of an underlying chronic disease, or of asymptomatic young adults, after initial assessment is warranted. In short, no matter how attractive the instrument or how easy its administration, its use for all patients at every visit is not recommended.

Disease-Specific Functional Assessment

Patients visit their physicians for a variety of reasons but discomfort from illness ranks high among those reasons. Usually, physicians evaluate symptoms, physical findings, and laboratory results to make a diagnosis, or when a diagnosis cannot be made, a group of possible diagnostic entities that can explain the findings. Screening for either undetected disease or functional impairment is not an integral part of this process and, therefore, is frequently neglected. If physicians are to incorporate functional assessment into daily practice, a rational insertion of this into patient care will be required.

Functional status assessment should be integrated into the recording of the several components of the clinical encounter. Recording should be episode and problem oriented, with linkage of components to each other as follows: reason for encounter → process items (examination, laboratory work-up, X-ray) → diagnosis → functional assessment → process items (therapy, drugs, etc.). Periodic functional status assessments are recommended for all persons with chronic diseases. They are not recommended for episodes of acute self-limited illnesses unless there is an underlying chronic disease that could be exacerbated by these episodes or unless these episodes of illness persist for more than six weeks. Depending upon the nature of the disease, initial assessment may be made with the same tools that are used for screening or with more complex measurements designed for specified functional deficits. Time intervals between assessments will depend upon the type of the disease and its severity.

An example of how clinical indicators and functional status assessment can be incorporated into a health problem rubric of the *ICHPPC-2-Defined* (8) is given for hypertension.

Uncomplicated hypertension, primary or secondary including hypertension NOS; labile hypertension
Note: if secondary hypertension, code for underlying cause

Inclusion in this rubric requires both of the following:

1. Either (i) two or more readings per encounter, taken at two or more encounters, for blood pressures that average over 95 mm Hg diastolic or over 160 mm Hg systolic in adult patients or (ii) two or more readings at a single encounter with an average diastolic blood pressure of 120 mm Hg or more.
2. Absence of evidence of secondary involvement of heart, kidney, or brain due to hypertension.

It is suggested that the following be periodically assessed: (i) blood pressure; (ii) kidney function with urine protein, blood urea nitrogen, and creatinine; (iii) heart function with electrocardiogram and/or echocardiogram; (iv) cerebrovascular status with fundus examination; and (v) overall function with the Dartmouth COOP charts.

The many chronic health problems that require specification of specific clinical end points plus overall functional status assessment include the following from *ICHPPC-2-Defined*:

Chapter   1. Infective and parasitic diseases
                 Tuberculosis, postherptic neuragliga
Chapter   2. Neoplasms
                 All neoplasms

Chapter 3. Endocrine
          Diabetes mellitus, gout, obesity
Chapter 4. Blood diseases
          Pernicious anemia
Chapter 5. Mental disorders
          All mental disorders
Chapter 6. Nervous system disorders
          Multiple sclerosis, epilepsy, Parkinson's disease
Chapter 7. Circulatory system diseases
          Chronic ischemic heart disease, heart failure, hypertension
Chapter 8. Respiratory system diseases
          Pleural effusion, emphysema, chronic obstructive pulmonary
          disease
Chapter 9. Digestive system diseases
          Duodenal ulcer, irritable bowel syndrome
Chapter 10. Genitourinary system diseases
          Chronic pyelonephritis, prostatitis, menopausal symptoms
Chapter 11. Pregnancy
Chapter 12. Skin diseases
          Psoriasis, alpecia
Chapter 13. Musculoskeletal diseases
          Osteoarthritis, back pain osteoporosis
Chapter 14. Congenital anomalies
          All congenital anomalies
Chapter 16. Signs, symptoms
          All that persist longer than six weeks
Chapter 17. Trauma
          All with late effects
Chapter 18. Supplementary
          All social, mental, and family problems

Although the above list is far from complete, the task of providing specific clinical end points and functional assessments for each disease is formidable. Yet, the WONCA Classification Committee builds on an impressive amount of preliminary work, not the least of which are the inclusion and exclusion criteria for the many health problems in the *ICHPPC-2-Defined*.

Several problems, nevertheless, remain:

1. Determining which of several functional status assessment instruments are best suited to assess disease-specific changes;
2. demonstrating high degrees of validity and reliability of these instruments in the ambulatory care settings within many countries; and
3. reaching an agreement on the most appropriate clinical end points as well as their quantification.

The goals, however, are important and can be achieved. The committee, therefore, has no choice but to continue this important work.

Conclusions

Functional status assessment is both desirable and feasible in the ambulatory care setting. These assessments should be made a part of screening, as well as linked to specific diseases. For this purpose several functional status assessment instruments may be required. If the major objective is to assess outcome, the objective recording of signs, symptoms, and laboratory results, in addition to functional status assessment, will be required. Validity, reliability, and cross-cultural comparisons are needed for each instrument that is adopted. A method of incorporating functional status assessment into everyday practice and its interdigitation with the several WONCA classifications is suggested.

References

1. Jagger C, Clarke H. Mortality risks in the elderly: Five-year follow-up of total population. *Int J Epidemiol* 17:111–114, 1988.
2. Parkerson GR Jr, Gelbach SH, Wagner EH, et al. The Duke–UNC health profile: An adult health status instrument for primary care. *Med Care* 19:306–828, 1981.
3. Gilson BS, Gilson JS, Bergner M, et al. The sickness impact profile: Development of an outcome measure of health care. *Am J Public Health* 65:1304, 1975.
4. Fitts W. *Manual: Tennessee Self-Concept Scale.* Nashville, TN: Counselor Recordings and Tests, 1964.
5. Zung, WW. A self-rating depression scale. *Arch Gen Psych* 12:63, 1965.
6. West SR, Harris BJ, Warren A, et al. Terminal care: A retrospective study of patients with cancer in their terminal year. *New Zeal Med J* 99:197–200, 1986.
7. Nelson E, Wasson J, Kirk J, Keller A, et al. Assessment of function in routine clinical practice: Description of the COOP Chart Method and preliminary findings. *J Chron Dis* 40: (suppl 1):5S–63S, 1987.
8. WONCA Classification Committee. *ICHPPC-2-Defined* (International Classification of Health Problems in Primary Care), ed 3. Oxford, Oxford University Press, 1983.
9. WONCA Classification Committee. *IC-Process-PC* (International Classification of Process in Primary Care). Oxford, Oxford University Press, 1986.
10. Lamberts H, Wood M. *ICPC* (International Classification of Primary Care). Oxford, Oxford University Press, 1987.
11. WONCA Classification Committee. An international glossary for primary care. *J Fam Pract* 13:671–681.
12. Meenan RF, Gertman PM, Mason JH. Measuring health status in arthritis. The Arthritic Impact Measurement Scales. *Arthritis Rheum* 23:146–152, 1980.
13. Melzack R. The McGill Pain Questionnaire: Major properties and scoring methods, Pain 1:277–299, 1975.

6
Functional Status Assessment in Relation to Health Promotion and Preventive Medicine

C. BRIDGES-WEBB and J. BARRAND

There is now an understanding that health involves more than the absence of disease and that measuring health includes a much wider spectrum of considerations than morbidity alone. This is reflected in the headings of the main chapters of a recent book, *Measuring Health: A Guide to Rating Scales and Questionnaires* (1): "Functional Disability and Handicap," "Psychological Well-Being," "Social Health," Quality of Life and Life Satisfaction," Pain Measurements," and "General Health Measurements."

The wide spectrum of concepts that is included in rating scales and questionnaires for measuring health should also be applied to the somewhat different process of assessing functional status in medical care, so that assessment includes fitness, psychological well-being, and social functioning, as well as the extent of morbidity.

Evaluating outcomes of medical care requires that the goals set for each patient are measurable within an appropriate time scale. The goals need to include elements across the wide spectrum of health concepts in order to allow for the enormous variability between patients. To the extent that measurable goals can be standardized, audit or research involving comparisons of outcomes become possible. This would allow what Robert Westbury (personal communication) so well described as a "broad sweep continuous recording, without which GP studies could never offer the opportunistic insights into the real world" that they do.

Evaluation of outcomes of health promotion and preventive medicine requires techniques that are different from the usual process of clinical assessment. To the extent that health is compromised at the time, assessment of clinical status may allow subsequent reassessment at a later date as a measure of outcome. Examples would be improved excercise tolerance, more satisfying sleep patterns, or reduction in blood pressure. Such assessments are rather limited in two ways. First, they relate mainly to the physiological dimension of functioning. Second, although they can measure change from bad to good, it is difficult to measure change from good to better. A broader assessment of functional status, such as the COOP chart (2) provides, does allow improvement to be measured in terms of overall condition and change in social and emotional health, without necessarily presupposing initial abnormalities, and therefore goes some way towards meeting the need.

Resources for Health

Another way of assessing status in relation to health promotion and preventive medicine is to consider the individual's resources for health as modified from the suggestions of Antonovsky (3). These can, for convenience, be related to the three dimensions of functioning: physiological, intrapersonal, and social (Table 6.1) (4).

TABLE 6.1. Resources for health.

Physiological
1. Genetic
2. Constitutional
     age and sex
     nutrition
     body mass
     excercise
     immune status
     use of drugs
     medical conditions past and present
3. Intelligence and knowledge
     general
     about health and disease
     sources of information
     expectations
4. Preventive orientation
     husbanding of resources
     attitude towards risk taking
5. Material
     food
     shelter
Intrapersonal
1. Ego Identity
2. Commitment and control
3. Intimate relationships
Social
1. Group memberships
2. Continuance and cohesion
3. Coping strategies
4. Social belief systems
     Institutional—religion
     Intellectual—philosophy
     Phenomenological—magic
     Sensual—art
5. Cultural stability—roles
                    —rules
                    —rituals
                    —values

Assessing resources for health and planning to enhance them is much more feasible than trying to determine the extent to which individuals are healthy or even how well they are functioning.

Physiological Functioning

Assessment of physiological functioning relates to a number of the following resources:

Genetic make-up, which has much to do with size (height and weight), allergic diathesis, blood pressure, and predisposition to inherited and familial diseases;

constitutional factors, such as age, sex, nutrition, body mass, amount of excercise, use of drugs, immune status, vision and hearing, and past and present medical conditions;

knowledge, both general and about health and disease, sources of medical information, and health expectations;

Preventive orientation, ability, and willingness to husband resources and provide for future contingencies, and attitude towards risk taking;

material resources such as shelter, food, and money.

An assessment of genetic make-up involves taking a family medical history. In addition to general questions about diseases that run in the family and age and cause of death of parents and siblings, specific inquiries should be directed to a past or family history of the following:

allergies—hay fever, asthma, urticaria, and eczema;
diabetes
cancer of the breast and of the colon;
epilepsy;
gout;
glaucoma;
mental disorders, depression, and suicide; and
hypertension, heart disease, and stroke.

Such a history directs attention to areas of higher than usual risk for the patient.

Assessment of such constitutional factors as past and present medical condition and use of medication will be a routine part of the medical history, which should also cover the following:

allergies to food, drugs, or other substances;
immunization status and the possible need for booster injections;
nutritional assessment;
exercise;
use of alcohol, tobacco, caffeine, and other drugs; and
residence or work (past or present) in risk areas, for example, the tropics and dusty occupations, respectively.

The routine physical examination should be especially in areas indicated by the history but it should also include the following:

body mass index (M/H^2), where H is height in meters, and M is weight in kilograms. This should be between 20 and 25;
visual acuity, using a Snellen chart;
hearing, and inspection of ear for wax;
blood pressure;
mouth and teeth;
urinalysis;
body movements, gait, mobility, dexterity;
breasts in women; and
skin lesions.

Unless especially indicated by history or risk factors, special investigations are not often indicated as part of a routine assessment. Those that should most often be considered are

Pap smear in women every three years;
serum cholesterol and triglycerides at ages 30, 40, and 50 years; and
mammogram in women over 50 every year.

Assessment of the extent of the patient's knowledge about health and disease, their access to and use of sources of information, and their preventive orientation is rarely part of the clinical examination or of most measures of health. Since these factors may be important relative to motivation for change in life-style and health behavior, their evaluation should receive more attention.

Intrapersonal Functioning

Assessment of the patient as a person and the extent to which rapport can be established with the patient is important in evaluating the patient's ability to change.

Patients' commitment to life can be assessed relative to activities at work and at home, and leisure activities. Their sense of control over their own life (essential to motivation for change) should be determined. Anxiety and depression are commonly associated with a sense of lack of control. Patients asked directly about their sense of control are often surprised but are usually well able to respond with significant information, which is often more helpful than the answers to more standard questions, though these may still need to be asked:

1. Have you any life goals?
2. Do you like your job or daily routine?
3. Do you have intimate family or friends in whom you can confide?
4. Are your personal relationships satisfying?

5. Do you often let people you are intimate with know of your appreciation of them? Do you listen carefully to them?
6. Do you get enough relaxation and sleep?

Such an approach often leads naturally to sharing feelings about intimate relationships and sexuality. All these matters are of great significance in setting goals for health.

Social Functioning

Assessment of social functioning usually accompanies assessment of intrapersonal functioning. The patient's membership in groups, such as family, friends, work, and recreational groups will indicate the level of social support. Experiences of cohesion, being part of a society based on regularity and laws (formal and informal), and of continuance, being part of the flow of history, will relate much to group membership.

Coping strategies to deal with difficulties in life are often patterns for future behavior and need to be elicited. There can be elicited by asking such questions as

Who supports whom, and how?
To what extent do coping strategies include tobacco, alcohol, caffeine, and other drugs?
Has other medical help been used, and if so, how effective has it been? If it was not effective, why not?
Is the patient undergoing therapy, if so, in what area?
Is the patient using medication, and for what purpose?

Social belief systems, religion, philosophy, magic, and art may be significant; and the roles, rules, rituals, and values of the patient's culture need to be appreciated, even more when the patient's cultural background is different from the doctor's.

Establishing this background for understanding may in fact take place in the course of obtaining information about physiological functioning. However, unless it is held specifically in mind, it will often not proceed far enough to engender patient confidence.

Reassurance

Reassurance is an important part of the outcome of any checkup. Reassurance cannot be dispensed, it must develop in the patient. It does not develop unless the patient is confident that the doctor knows enough about the situation to understand it. Such confidence is related as much or more to understanding the patient's intrapersonal and social functioning as to understanding physiological functioning, though of course the three are so interrelated that their separation is merely an arbitrary but convenient approach. There is therefore good reason to emphasize the importance of assessment of intrapersonal and social resources.

Assessment of Health Resources

Clinical assessment relative to health promotion, and preventive medicine, often includes much that has been covered above, although rarely is it systematized in the way suggested in Table 6.1. The emphasis is usually on physiological status.

The development of instruments to measure health status has emphasized psychological and social functioning as well as physiological functioning (rather than status) (1). Most of these measuring instruments were developed for research purposes and have little applicability in day-to-day health care. One measure developed for use in clinical situations is the COOP chart method (2).

The COOP charts were developed to cover a core set of functional dimensions and indicators of life quality for use in clinical practice by the

TABLE 6.2. Assessment of resources for health.

Resource	Clinical practice[a,b]	COOP chart[b]
Physiological		
Genetic	+ +	–
Constitutional	+ + +	Physical condition
	+ + +	Pain
Intelligence and knowledge	–	–
Prevention orientation	–	–
Material needs	+	–
Intrapersonal	+	Emotional condition
	–	Quality of life
Ego identity	–	–
Commitment and control	–	–
Intimate relationships	–	–
Social		
Group membership	+	Social support
	+	Social activities
	+	Daily work
Continuance and cohesion	–	–
Coping strategies	–	–
Social belief systems	–	–
Cultural stability	–	–
	+	Overall condition
	+	Change in condition

[a] + to + + +, extent to which usually assessed.
[b] –, usually not assesed.

Department of Community and Family Medicine, Dartmouth Medical School, New Hampshire. They consist of nine charts, each with a five-level scale. Four charts relate to function (physical condition, emotional condition, daily work, and social activities), four charts relate to quality of life (quality of life, overall condition, pain, and social support), and one chart relates to change over the past four weeks. They have been evaluated in a number of countries under a variety of clinical conditions with different kinds of patients, and their reliability and validity have been documented. They appear to be a useful extension to methods of patient assessment in general practice.

Comparison of the kind of information for assessment of health resources usually gathered in clinical practice with that covered by the COOP charts indicates the way in which use of the charts complements normal clinical practice to broaden the range of resources assessed (Table 6.2). The charts assess resources as well as functional status. It is apparent, however, that there are areas that are not covered by either normal clinical practice or by the COOP charts. These include some aspects of physiological function, as well as most of the subheadings under intrapersonal and social functioning. If, as we suggest, assessment of intrapersonal and social resources are important not only for health but also for reassuring and motivating patients to change, to be healthier, then greater attention needs to be paid to evaluating the extent to which patients have each of these resources. That is a task for the future.

References

1. McDowell I, Newell C. *Measuring Health: A Guide to Rating Scales and Questionnaires.* Oxford, Oxford University Press, 1987.
2. Nelson EC, Wasson JH, Kirk JW. Assessment of function in routine clinical practice: Description of the COOP chart method and preliminary findings. *J Chron Dis* 40(s1):555–635, 1987.
3. Antonovsky A. *Health Stress and Coping.* San Francisco: Jossey-Bass, 1979, 184p.
4. Barrand J. A model of health. *Australian Family Physician* 14:1302–1307, 1985.

7
A Clinical Measure for Evaluating Patient Functioning in Diabetics

R.W. ELFORD, R.T. CONNIS, T.R. TAYLOR, M.J. GORDON, J.E. LILJENQUIST, R.S. MECKLENBERG, J.W. STEPHENS, and M. BAKER

Introduction

Many clinicians have noted that the clinical course of patients with chronic diseases that require long-sustained interventions is often characterized by discrepancies between their biomedical state and their capacity to function in a variety of roles. More recently, several clinicians have commented on the difficulty of interpreting and applying in clinical practice the results of many conventional therapeutic trials because of the lack of information about the patient's functional status. Both situations suggest the need for an approach to measure the impact of treatments on patients in a manner that qualitatively expands traditional biomedical outcomes.

This chapter evaluates the clinical use of a battery of patient-functioning measures, consisting of five different, relatively independent dimensions, on a sample of type-1 diabetic subjects. By employing a nonequivalent matched control group design for the diabetic subjects, we were able to show the adaptation to a change in treatment also: namely, the impact of commencing insulin infusion therapy on the various dimensions of patient functioning. A diabetic's ability to adapt to the insulin pump is demonstrated by a stabilization, a restoration, or an improvement in his/her serial patient functioning profiles. Predictably, we found a wide variability of functional status among patients. A notable profile pattern in younger diabetic patients was a higher incidence of poor adaptation in their emotional, social, and cognitive areas of functioning.

This approach to evaluating the impact of the insuline pump by measuring serial changes in patient functioning has many generic features that could qualitatively expand the clinical assessment of other new medical technologies in therapeutic trials.

The Literature

Diabetes literature over the past decade has suggested a causal link between chronic hyperglycemia and long-term microvascular complications, particularly retinal, renal, and myocardial lesions (1,2). Accordingly, diabetes management regimens involving intensified metabolic control have been emphasized as a means of delaying or preventing long-term complications.

Although there has been a failure to substantiate the long-term benefits of tight control regimens (3, 4), the clinical utilization of intensified regimens featuring insulin delivery by automated pumps, multiple daily injections, and home glucose monitoring is broadening the hope that such regimens will prove to be efficacious. However, the long-term efficacy of such regimens may, ultimately, require patient compliance and an ability to adapt personally and psychologically to the rigid demands inherent in maintaining glucose control.

To date, studies have found improvements in blood glucose levels within a few hours or days after initiation of intensive insulin infusion therapy, with few adverse side effects of note (5–7). However, other studies of longer duration suggest that the regimen presents unique, longer-term problems to both the patient and the physician. In addition to regular maintenance activities such as battery charging, home glucose monitoring, and frequent communication with the physician, the patient must deal indefinitely with possible injection site inflammation, tube blockages, or delivery system malfunction (8). Short-term and cross-sectional studies have been important in establishing the efficacy of the insulin pump regimen, and in showing that no deterioration in levels of depression, self-esteem, or social adjustment take place (9). However, the lack of adverse side effects reported in these studies seems incongruent with the large reported dropout rates among insulin pump users (ranging from 20 to 80%) (6, 10, 11).

An explanation for the large dropout rate of pump users may lie in the personal activities involved in the maintenance of the regimen and/or in the loss of capacity to derive satisfaction from a variety of roles in day-to-day life (12). Longer-term longitudinal research is needed to critically examine the impact of the insulin pump (an intrusive intervention) on patient functioning.

During the interval of time between the development of a new efficacious intervention and its general adoption by health practitioners as an effective treatment, each therapeutic regimen must be assessed for its contribution to the major tasks of medical care, namely, curing the disease, prolonging life, and enhancing the quality of life (13).

With the emergence of new methods of measuring health status, clinical assessment of the quality of life of patients has now become more feasible. Assessments of functional status before and after the application of a new treatment can provide a broader, more objective measure of the treatment impact (14, 15). Additionally, determining patient functional status with a systems perspective before the initiation of a treatment may be a useful way to predict the patient's response to a particular treatment alternative (16).

Ware (17), using a multilevel systems perspective based on proximity to disease-specific functional status, defined five relatively independent levels of health status and disease impact:

1. Disease specific indicators (biomedical test)
2. Physical functioning (activities of daily living)

3. Emotional functioning (distress/well-being)
4. Social functioning (performance of social roles)
5. General health perceptions

After an exhaustive review of the literature, we have concluded that this systems model for assessing functional status could provide an approach for evaluating the impact of a clinical intervention. Because type 1 diabetes mellitus requires a fairly specific intervention (insulin), assessment of the impact of different insulin regimens appeared to be an appropriate disease model in which to evaluate our approach to measuring functional status.

Methods

Measurement of Patient Functioning

Clinically, assessing how well a patient is functioning often can be a difficult and lengthy process. Standardized questionnaires designed to provide a broader base of information about functional ability in ambulatory patients would be an attractive supplement to clinical assessment. Under circumstances in which an investigator requires more objective data in order to estimate the burden/advantage of a new therapeutic regimen, systematic recording of functional status is important. Many valid, reliable measurement instruments that have multidimensional indices and separate subscales are available; they are quantifiable, sensitive, and stable over serial assessments and can be either self-administered or telephone administered (18, 19).

After a thorough review of the appropriateness, utility, validity, and reliability of numerous instruments and after a discussion with clinical consultants, the study group developed a battery of instruments designed to assess each of the functional dimensions proposed by Ware. Table 7.1 is a summary of the complete instrument package.

TABLE 7.1. Measures for study of patient functioning.

Dimension	Name of instrument	Average time for completion (minutes)
1	Glycosylated hemoglobin—quaterly (colormetric method on frozen samples)	
	Fasting blood glucose—monthly diary —medical record	
2	Duke–UNC Health Profile	10
	Pump problem checklist	5
3	Spielberger state—trait anxiety	5
	Profile of mood states	5
	Rand Mental Health Inventory	5
4	Health and daily living form (Moos)	10
5	Rand general health perceptions index	5
	DCCT quality of life questionnaire	10
	Health locus of control	5

Determination of Optimal Measurement Indicator for Each Dimension

Two approaches were employed to select the set of indicators that most rigorously predicted functional status—a correlational model and a factor analysis model. The former requires fewer instruments and has a simpler analysis, the latter is methodologically more rigorous and is more precise.

Correlational Model

An intercorrelation matrix containing the variables (Table 7.1) that contributed to each dimension was constructed. The variable that correlated most highly with the other variables was chosen as the indicator for that dimension. Table 7.2 displays the indicator (a numerical score derived from a single instrument) selected to represent each dimension.

Factor Analysis Model

Confirmatory factor analysis was performed for three of the five different dimensions using the maximum likelihood procedures of the LISREL V program. The remaining two dimensions (disease-specific indicator and general health perception) were represented by only a single measure. The measured indicators for each dimension were selected based upon their content validity, and the total factor model was examined for goodness of fit. Variables with factor loadings below a certain criterion were dropped until a model was found that best explained the covariation of variables. The scrore for each factor is an algorithmic function of the factor weights and the standardized Z-score transformation for the indicators within each dimension.

TABLE 7.2. Indicators for each dimension.

Dimension	Name of indicator
1	Disease-specific indicators: 30-day fasting glucose mean (20)
2	Physical functioning: — from Health and Daily Living Form (21) medical conditions and symptoms
3	Emotional functioning: — from Rand Corp. (22) distress/well-being (MHI-9)
4	Social functioning: — from Health and Daily Living Form (23) social activities with family and friends
5	General Health Perceptions: — from Rand Corp (24) general health perception index

The derived factor structure was then cross-validated on another group of type 1 diabetics in either an intensified control insulin regime or a conventional management regime. Table 7.3 portrays the combination of indicator scores found to be most predictive for each of the different dimensions. Each dimension of patient functioning can, therefore, be represented by a single factor score. Table 7.3 shows the percent of variability explained by the factor score in each dimension (coefficient of determination). Measures listed in boldface type indicate variable(s) found within each dimension that contributed most to the factor score for that dimension.

A comparison of the two models demonstrates that the two approaches provide qualitatively similar results, and that they lead to similar clinical interpretations. For the purposes of this chapter, the shorter, more practical correlational model was utilized for the demonstration of the clinical application of our assessment approach because it appeared to be methodologically acceptable when compared to the factor analysis model.

TABLE 7.3. Predictive indicator for each dimension.

Dimension	Name of Instrument	Coefficient of determination
1	Disease-specific indicators: —30-days fasting mean (20)	100%
2	Physical functioning: —from Duke–UNC Health Profile (24) —**Duke symptoms** —Duke personal functioning —from Health and Daily Living Form (21) —HDL symptoms —HDL medical condition —HDL medication use	83%
3	Emotional functioning: —from Rand Corp. (23) —**Distress (MHI-7)** —Well-being (MHI-8) —from Health and Daily Living Form (21) —HDL-11, global depression —from Speilberger State–Trait Anxiety Inventory (25) —State anxiety —from Duke–UNC Health Profile (24) —Duke-4, emotional functioning	93%
4	Social functioning: —from Health and Daily Living Form (21) —**close circle of friends** —number of close relationships —number of friends —social activities with friends	68%
5	General Health Perceptions: —from Rand Corp. (23) —**General Health Perception Index**	100%

SUBJECTS

After selecting a chronic disease (type 1 diabetes mellitus) with substantial diversity of patient functioning, and after choosing a model for assessing the impact of change in treatments (Ware's Health status, and Disease Impact), a sample of diabetic patients was studied in order to determine the clinical-usefulness of our measure of patient functioning.

An extensive data set from a larger research project that assessed the functional status of type 1 diabetic patients on three different insulin regimes (conventional, intensive insulin, pump infusion) provided the required sample (26–28). Patients for the larger study were obtained from primary and specialist care facilities in the Pacific Northwest, representing care for a large number of insulin therapy patients in Washington, Oregon, Idaho, and Montana. Subjects were screened to determine whether they met the following inclusion criteria: (i) medical documentation of type 1 diabetes mellitus (ii) 17 to 55 years of age, (iii) no complications that would preclude participation, (iv) not pregnant, and (v) undergoing regular followup checks at least every 3 months by a physician with training and experience in the management of diabetics.

For this chapter, data concerning two groups of subjects were analyzed: (i) a pump group—35 type 1 diabetic patients who had initiated insulin infusion pump therapy, within the past year and (ii) a conventional group—50 type 1 diabetic patients on conventional insulin therapy. Each pump patient had been matched with one or more conventional patients for such characteristics as age, sex, number of diabetic complications, and duration of diabetes.

STUDY DESIGN

The data set analyzed for this chapter employed a nonequivalent control group design, and utilized serial assessment of the two groups across a 12-month period. The data collected allowed (i) longitudinal descriptions of individual subjects, (ii) analyses of cross-sectional differences between groups at various points in time, and (iii) longitudinal analyses of repeated measures (over a minimum of a 12-month window). This chapter reports on selected aspects arising from all three modes of analysis and focuses on the impact of insulin infusion pump therapy on the various dimensions of functioning in type 1 diabetic patients.

GRAPHIC DISPLAY OF PATIENT FUNCTIONING MEASURES

A means of displaying the entire profile of patient functioning consisting of all five dimensions was devised as follows:

1. Normative data and descriptive statistics for the population used for the development of each instrument were obtained by reviewing the publications and technical reports for each of the measurement intruments.

2. Descriptive statistics for the conventional and pump groups in the diabetic sample of this project were calculated, cross sectionally.
3. Statistical tests for differences between the general population and study sample (Z-test) and between the pump and conventional sample groups (T-test) were performed.

The standardized indicator score, which represented the highest intercorrelation among variables within a given dimension, was calculated for the diabetic sample, using the population normative data and the study sample statistics of a Z-score transformation. At this stage, an individual's standardized score from each dimension can be plotted against a "normative background" derived from both the general population and the diabetic sample.

Finally, using a simple algorithm, each individual's raw instrument scores were transformed by a microcomputer program to scores that could be plotted against a normative background that was derived from the diabetic sample and displayed as a chart. The microcomputer-generated summary bar graph allows an individual's profile to be compared to a normative range of individuals. In this profile, on each dimension zero (0) indicates the general population score. If over time an individual's score moves towards zero (0), it indicates an improvement in functioning.

Results

The distribution by age for the two groups of interest here ranged from 17 to 47 years, with the majority of subjects being in their 20s or 30s. The male/female ratio was 1/1. No significant differences between the conventional group and the pump group were found on age, sex, duration of diabetes, or number of medical complications. Further comparisons using such demographic and clinical variables as marital status, education, employment status, nondiabetes-related medical problems, and medication use yielded only one difference between groups—their blood sugar goals. [The pump group reported significantly lower blood sugar goals than the conventional group (30, 31).] In general pretest comparisons of patient functioning suggested that the conventional and pump groups were highly similar but not identical.

Two normative ranges are referred to in this study: the "general population" and the "diabetic sample." Each was standardized with a Z-transformation. Comparison of the general population with the diabetic sample standardized scores resulted in the observation that the diabetic sample significantly differed from the general population on all dimensions except emotional functioning. [The Z-test value in the Z-test column of Table 7.4 is well above the significance level (2.00) in all dimensions except for the MHI-9 pump group.] Comparison of the pump sample with the conventional sample resulted in the observation that the two samples are similar in all dimensions

TABLE 7.4. Comparison of normative data for several population and diabetic sample.

Dimension	Instrument	N	Sample[a]	Mean	S.D.	Z-test	T-test	Z-score S.D.	Z-score Mean	Z-score Low	Z-score High
Biomedical	FBS	1,446	gen. pop	93.55	15.34	23		5	3.9	2.9	4.9
		35	diabetic	154.4	76.7						
Physical	HDLI	424	gen. pop.	2.72	1.89			1.25	1.3	0	2.6
		35	pump	5.17	2.36	10	0.9				
		1446	conv.	5.58		9.5					
	HDL2	424	gen. pop.	2.25	2.54						
		35	pump	3.34	3.09	2.54	0.91				
		50	conv.	3.98	3.34	4.81					
Emotional	MH19	5089	gen. pop.	177.6	25.46			1.1	-0.23	-1.4	0.9
		35	pump	179	30.08	0.335	2.32				
		50	conv.	164.3	26.6	3.67					
Social	HDL30	424	gen. pop.	10.2	2.82			0.79	-0.8	-1.6	0
		35	pump	8.03	2.35	1.77	0.4				
		50	conv.	8.22		1.59					
	HDL31	424	gen. pop.	5.38	2.79						
		35	pump	4.04	2.29	3.39	0.04				
		50	conv.	4.04	2.42	3.39					
GHP	GHP7	4717	gen. pop.	83.36	13.54			1.15	-0.93	-2.1	0.22
			pump	73.79	15.54	4.18	1.63				
			conv.	68.32	14.86	7.85					

[a]Gen., general; Pop., population; Conv., conventional.

except for biomedical (the pump group had lower blood sugars) and emotional functioning (the pump group had higher scores). [The T-test value in the T-test column in Table 7.4 is below the significance level (1.96) in all dimensions except the MHI-9 diabetic sample.]

Clinical Case Applications

Several illustrative case profiles derived from the sample of type 1 diabetic patients in this study are shown in Figures 7.1 and 7.4 and are used to demonstrate the utility and application of this methodology. The background range in the figures for each dimension of the profile was constructed from the diabetic sample descriptive statistics displayed in the three Z-score columns (lower, mean, and upper) of Table 7.4. The "light" background range in the profiles represents one standard deviation about the mean score for the diabetic sample. The midpoint, or mean, of this range is shifted away from zero (general population mean) in the direction and to the amount that the diabetic sample is different from that of the general population. Individual scores were derived from the case statistics in Table 7.5, and are represented by the dark superimposed bars.

The scale has been standardized, with zero representing the normative mean. Therefore, more normal functioning is portrayed by scores that are approaching zero.

CASE NO. 1

Figures 7.1 and 7.2 show the base-line and 12-month profiles of a 21-year-old woman who is married, who works as a medical secretary, and who was diagnosed as a type 1 diabetic (16) years ago (No. 318). This patient demonstrates an ideal pattern of adaptation to her insulin pump. Her base-line profile, as displayed in Figure 7.1, shows poor biomedical control, several physical problems, a depressed emotional state, limited social functioning, and a below-average general health perception index.

Her 12-month profile, shown in Figure 7.2, shows improved scores in every dimension, her individual score has moved into the normative range for the diabetic sample. Her dramatically improved biomedical and physical functioning has been accompained by more normal scores on the other three dimensions. Unfortunately, such an ideal pattern of adaptation was rarely found in the diabetic sample of this study.

CASE NO. 2

The opposite type of pattern, representing poor adaptation, is shown in Figures 7.3 and 7.4. This 36-year-old male is married, works as a salesman, and was diagnosed as a type 1 diabetic 12 years ago (No. 316).

His base-line profile, as displayed in Figure 7.3, looks ideal for an infusion pump candidate. All dimensions, except the biomedical, are well within the

TABLE 7.5. Individual scores for various dimensions of patent functioning.

Case scores					Biomedical			Physical		
CASE #	Age	Sex	Demographic	duration	base	6 mon	12 mon	base	6 mon	12 mon
316 r	36	m	salesman, married	12 yr.	203		265	3	5	3
z			16 yr. ed		7		11	0.15	1.2	0.15
318 r	21	f	med. sec. married	16 yr.	279.6	151.5	122	12	7	4
z			13 yr. ed		12	3.8	2	4.9	2.3	0.7

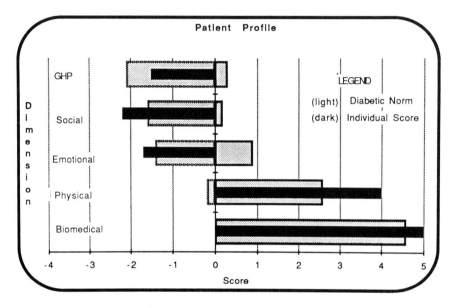

FIGURE 7.1. Base-line profile—case No. 1.*

*Zero (0) represents the general population average score, scores approaching 0 indicate good functioning, scores far away from 0 indicate poor functioning.

range of the diabetic sample, and indeed on three dimensions, the scores are very close to the general population average. One would anticipate that a more precise method for gaining biomedical control would meet this man's needs.

However, his functioning pattern dramatically changed after 12 months on the pump. Figure 7.4, shows that this patient continues to have poor biomedical control, and his emotional and social functioning appears to have deteriorated. Even more pronounced, however, is his general health perception score, which is well outside the diabetic sample range.

A detailed exploration of the overall impact of infusion therapy with this patient is needed to clarify the overall utility of his treatment regimen and to determine if there are any trade-offs that might lead to a less erratic profile.

TABLE 7.5. (Continued).

	Emotional			Social			GHP	
base	6 mon	12 mon	base	6 mon	12 mon	base	6 mon	12 mon
184	160	151	9	13	6	59	57	42
0.25	− 0.7	− 1	− 0.4	0.9	− 1.5	− 1.8	− 1.8	− 3
134	182	176	4	7	7	63	57	75
− 1.7	0.25	0	− 2.2	− 1.1	− 1.1	− 1.5	− 1.8	− 0.6

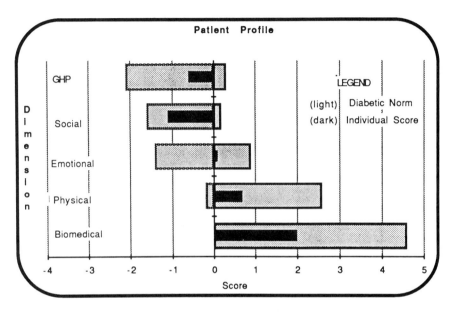

FIGURE 7.2. Twelve-month profile—case No. 1.*

*Zero (0) represents the general population average score, scores approaching 0 indicate good functioning, scores far away from 0 indicate poor functioning.

Conclusion

The design and measurement instruments employed in this study allow reliable comparison of individual profiles to those of the diabetic sample ($n = 85$) and to the normative statistics of the general population. As in other attempts to measure features of clinical medicine objectively, which have traditionally been left to clinical judgment, the profiles are useful only if they can increase the precision with which clinical decisions can be made. The biomedical benefits for insulin pump infusion therapy were readily demonstrated in early studies, and the initial reaction was to think that all insulin-dependent diabetics would benefit from this new technology. However, a

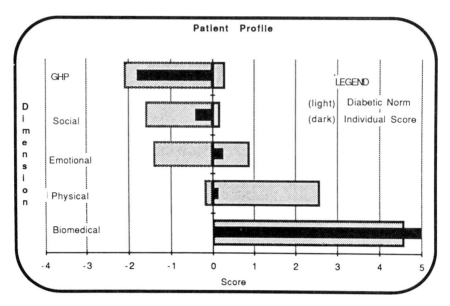

FIGURE 7.3. Base-line profile—case No. 2.*

*Zero (0) represents the general population average score, scores approaching 0 indicate good functioning, scores far away from 0 indicate poor functioning.

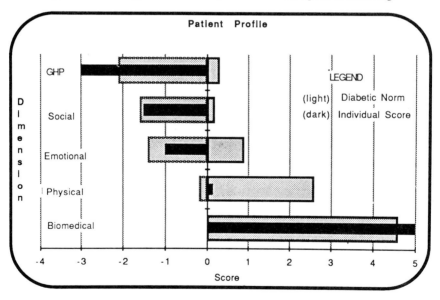

FIGURE 7.4. Twelve-month profile—case No. 2.*

*Zero (0) represents the general population average score, scores approaching 0 indicate good functioning, scores far away from 0 indicate poor functioning.

number of unanticipated problems were encountered, such as high dropout rates and little or no improvement in functional status. It appears that decision making about whether to employ insulin infusion therapy requires additional information on the part of the physician and the patient.

The wide variability of adaptation among patients on insulin pump infusion therapy can be better understood when it is described in the context of a model displaying the functional status of the patient. These statements about changes in functional status of individuals on pump therapy are only descriptive, and other events in an individual's life, such as marital stress, intercurrent illness, and change in job status, might have altered the data independent of the method of diabetes therapy. Because the pretest comparisons on demographic and clinical variables yielded no significant group differences between the conventional and pump groups, we would anticipate that such life changes would have a similar likelihood of occurring in either group. For certain individuals, however, the combination of life events and a stringent regimen may create observable dysfunction in their profiles, thereby alerting the clinician that a reassessment of their regimen is in order.

The cohort design and sample size are not sufficient to make causal inferences; however, several patterns appear to suggest an association of the institution and maintenance of insulin pump therapy and some adverse reactions among younger patients. The clinical relevance of these patterns, in terms of predicting dropouts, patient satisfaction, and successful adaptation, awaits further validation, perhaps by utilizing the methodology employed in this study. The trade-offs that may need to be made in terms of different dimensions of functioning are sufficiently well elucidated to allow discussions of those areas with the patient prior to commencing insulin infusion therapy. Often such focused communication can avert potential problems and lead to better adaptation to a new management approach.

This systems model of assessing functional impact may be used by physicians as a way of broadening their disease-specific perspective, as well as a method of corroborating their own clinical judgments. This method, combined with the existing technology, could pave the way for a better standardized, holistic approach to clinical medicine.

Clinicians interpreting impact patterns from this systems model would be able to obtain a qualitative understanding of the patient, and an estimate of the advantages of treatment, far beyond those gleaned from flow sheets containing only conventional biomedical data. With a little additional effort, we can readily obtain measurement instruments to be completed by the patient; then the raw scores may be entered into an applications program for a microcomputer, which, in turn, prints out the patient's profile on a graph to allow comparison of the patient with a normative range of patients, derived by statistical methods. Because many features of patient functioning are not disease-specific, this methodology may have a generic nature that can also be used to assess the impact of other new medical technologies.

A systems-oriented measurement model has been proposed in this study to assist in quantifying subjective clinical impressions that may often be observed when assessing the clinical impact of a new technology in medicine. This correlational model of patient functioning, with the various dimensions of functional status, can also be employed to expand the assessment of efficacy and effectiveness of new medical technologies qualitatively. By using profiles as a monitoring device, an investigator can see at a glance areas of poor function relative to a normative range. Finally, a clinician can explore the profile in detail with the patient and consider the functional trade-offs among the various dimensions that must be made in order to achieve particular biomedical goals.

Acknowledgments. This work at the Department of Family Medicine at the University of Washington was supported by the Robert Wood Johnson Foundation (grant∗8230).

We wish to thank the collaborating physicians who contributed patients to the study: from Pocatello—M. Baker: from Idaho Falls—J.E. Liljenquist; from Tacoma—D. McKowen; from Spokane—C. Carey, B. Gould, and J. Hartman; from Portland—J.W. Stephens, O.C. Page, R.L. Hare, C.S. Belknap, R.D. Hohl, R.C. and Biesbroeck; from Mason Clinic, Seattle—R.S. Mecklenburg, E.A. Bensoon, J.W. Benson, P.N. Frelund, R.J. Metz, and R.L. Nielson.

We gratefully acknowledge the contribution of the Clinical Management Research Group team.

References

1. Cahill GF, Etzwiler DD, et al.: Blood glucose control in diabetes. *Diabetes* 25:237–239, 1976.
2. Tchobroutsky G: Relation of diabetes control to development of microvascular complications. *Diabetologia* 15:143–152, 1978.
3. Pirart A: Diabetes mellitus and its degenerative complications: A prospective study of 4000 patients observed between 1947 and 1973. *Diabetes Care* 1:168–187, 1978.
4. Ainslie MB: Why tight diabetes control should be approached with caution. *Diabetes Control*, 75(4):49–53. 1984.
5. Seigler DE, La Greca A, et al.: Psychological effects of intensification of diabetic control. *Diabetes Care* 5(suppl 1):19–23, 1982.
6. Shapiro J, Wigg D, et al.: Personality and family profiles of chronic insulin dependent diabetic patients using conventional and portable insulin infusion therapy. *Diabetes Care* 7(2):137–142, 1984.
7. Marliss EB, Caron D: Present and future expections regarding insulin infusion pumps. *Diabetes Care* 4(2):325–327, 1981.
8. Mecklenberg RS, Benson JW, et al.: Clinical use of the insulin infusion pump in 100 patients with type 1 diabetes. *New Engl J Med* 307(9):513–518, 1982.
9. Rudolf MC, Ahern JA, et al.: Optimal insulin delivery in adolescent diabetes.

Impact of intensive treatment on psychosocial adjstment. *Diabetes Care* 5(suppl. 1):53–57, 1982.

10. Deeb LC, Williams PE: Premature mortality from diabetes. *J Fl Med Assoc* 69(12):1004–1008, 1982.
11. Dupre J, Champion M: Advances in insulin delivery in the management of diabetes mellitus. *Clin Endocrinol Met* 11(2):525–548, 1982.
12. Dunn SM, Turtle JR: The myth of the diabetic personality. *Diabetes Care* 4:645, 1981.
13. Moses L, Brown B Wm: Experiences with evaluating and safety and efficacy of medical technologies. *Ann Rev Publ Health* 5:267–292, 1984.
14. Ware, J: Monitoring and evaluating health, a commentary. *Med Care* 23(5):705–709, 1985.
15. Wenger NK, Mattson ME, et al.: *Assessment of Quality of Life in Clinical Trials of Cardiovascular Therapies.* Le Jacq Publishing Inc, New York. USA, 1984.
16. Guyatt G, Bombardier C, Tugwell P: Measuring Disease-Specific Quality of Life in Clinical Trials. CMAJ, Apr. 1986; Vol. 134, 889–894.
17. Ware J: *Conceptualizing Disease Impact and Treatment Outcomes.* WD-1789-HHS, Rand Corporation Publication Service, Santa Monica, CA, Mar 1983.
18. Bergner M: Measurement of health status. *Med Care*, (5):696–704, 1985.
19. Jette A, Davies A, Cleary PD, Calkins DR, Rubinstein LV, Fink A, Kosecoff J, Young RT, Brook RH, Delbanco TL: The functional status questionnnaire: Reliability and validity when used in primary care. *J Gen Int Med* 1:143–149, 1986.
20. Sayetta RB, Murphy RS: Summary of current diabetes-related data from the National Center for Health Statistics. *Diabetes Care*, 105–119, 1979.
21. Moos RH, Cronkite RC, et al.: *Health and Daily Living Form Manual.* Palo Alto, CA, Social Ecology Laboratory, Verterans Administration and Stanford University Medical Centers, 1984.
22. Veit C, Ware J: The structure of psychological distress and well-being in general populations. *J Consult Clin Psychol* (5):730–742, 1983.
23. Davies AR, Ware JE: Measuring Health Perceptions in the Health Insurance Experiments. R-2711-HHs, Rand Publications Series, San Francisco, 1981.
24. Parkerson G, Gehlbach S, Wagner E, James SA, Clapp NE, Muhlbaier LH: The Duke–UNC Health Profile: An adult health status instrument for primary care. *Med Care* 19(8):806–823, 1981.
25. Speilberger CD, Gorsuch RL, et al.: *Manual for the State–Trait Anxiety Inventory* (self-evaluation questionnaire). Palo Alto, CA, Consulting Psychologists Press, 1970.
26. Connis RT, Gordon MJ, Taylor TR: Changes in cognitive and social functioning of diabetic patients following initiation of insulin infusion therapy. *Experimental Aging Res.* 15(2):51–60, 1989.
27. Mengel MB, Connis RT, Gordon MJ, Taylor TR: The relationship of family dynamics and social support to personal, psychological, social functioning in diabetic patients on the insulin pump. *Fam Systems Med.* 6(3):317–333, 1988.
28. Connis RT: *Age Related Changes in Functioning of Insulin Dependent Diabetic Patients: The Impact of Insulin Infusion Therapy on Development.* Doctoral dissertation, University of Washington, February, 1986.

Part III   Dartmouth COOP Charts

8
The COOP Function Charts: A System to Measure Patient Function in Physicians' Offices

E.C. NELSON, J.M. LANDGRAF, R.D. HAYS, J.W. KIRK, J.H. WASSON, A. KELLER, and M. ZUBKOFF

Introduction

This book is based on the premise that physicians need, but do not have, accurate and efficient methods for measuring a patient's overall functional health status. In this chapter we describe a very brief method for measuring function and health that may be useful for routine use in primary care settings. This method is called the COOP chart system. The COOP chart system has been tested in many different practices in different parts of the world. This chapter is the second published report on the validity, reliability, and acceptability of the COOP charts. The first was published in the March 1987 supplement to the *Journal of Chronic Disease* (1). Further information on the COOP charts is available from the authors.

The next section describes: (i) our design principles, (ii) the system we developed to measure functioning (i.e., the COOP chart system), (iii) the strategy used to evaluate the reliability, validity, acceptability, and utility of the system, and (iv) the characteristics of the settings in which the COOP charts were evaluated.

Design Principles

Many validated measures of health status are available (2), but the vast majority are not suitable for office practice because they require too much time to administer and score. The goal of the COOP was to develop a measure specifically for office practices that used only six design principles. The chart system should

Produce reliable and valid data on a core set of dimensions of functioning and well-being (e.g., physical functioning, role functioning, social functioning, and emotional status);
be acceptable to patients, physicians, and office staff;
be applicable to a wide range of problems and diagnoses;
possess a high degree of face validity;
yield easily interpretable scores; and

provide the practitioner with clinically useful information regarding patients' functioning and well-being.

Description of the COOP Chart System

Our approach is called the "COOP chart" system because it was developed by the Dartmouth COOP Project, a network of community practices that cooperate on research activities and because the scales used to measure function are each displayed on a different chart. At the heart of the COOP system are charts that measure physical, social, and role functioning; emotional status; and overall health. Additional charts were developed for use, based on (i) clinician interest in using the method to measure a particular health indicator (e.g., pain and change in health) or (ii) the researcher interest in using the chart strategy to measure other health-related measures (e.g., social support and quality of life). There are a total of nine charts in the current COOP system: three focus on specific dimensions of function, two relate to symptoms or feelings, three are concerned with perceptions, and one is a health covariate (Table 8.1).

The charts are similar to Snellen charts, which are used medically to measure visual acuity quickly. Each chart consists of a simple title, a straightforward question referring to the status of the patient over the past four weeks, and five response choices. Each response is illustrated by a drawing that depicts a level of functioning or well-being along a five-point ordinal scale. In accordance with clinical convention, high scores represent unfavorable levels of health (life quality or social support) on each respective chart. For example, physical chart responses range from 1 to 5 with a score of 5 representing major limitations. One chart, health change, is scored differently: in this case a value of 3 indicates no change, whereas a score of 5 indicates a change for the worse and 1 a change for the better. Appendix A reproduces the charts highlighted in this chapter.

Source of Chart Contents

There are many excellent methods for measuring function that preceded the development of the COOP charts. The charts were modeled after and built

TABLE 8.1. Dimensions measured by COOP charts.[a]

Functional	Symptoms/Feelings
Physical function (physical condition)	Pain
Role function (daily work)	Emotional status (emotional condition)
Social function (social activities)	
Perceptions	Health Covariate
Quality of life (quality of life)	Social support
Overall health (overall condition)	
Health change (change in condition)	

[a] The title used on each chart is shown in parentheses following the dimension it measures.

upon certain features of these forerunners. For example, the physical function chart is based on such classical work as the Katz activities of daily living (ADL) index (3) and the New York Heart Association's functional classification (4), as well as the Goldman Specific Activity Scale (5). These were all designed for use in medical practice and they are to easy to administer, score, and interpret. However, the ADL index is most appropriate for long-term–care patients with extensive limitations in physical functioning and is not appropriate for ambulatory patients who have higher levels of physical ability. The New York Heart Association's measure, although popular and easy to use, focuses on limitations due to heart problems and has been shown by Goldman to be unreliable. The emotional status chart was based on earlier research conducted by the COOP and on the mental health inventory developed at RAND (6, 7).

In other respects the charts resemble some of the best multidimensional measures of function such as the sickness impact profile (SIP) (8), the Duke–UNC Health Profile (9), the McMaster Health Index (10), the Nottingham Health Profile (11), and the health status measures developed by Ware and his colleagues at RAND (12). All of these measures are multidimensional (i.e., they assess physical, mental, and social function) and have been subjected to careful methodological studies to determine their reliability and validity.

In addition to using earlier instruments as a resource, content for the charts came from clinicians and health measurement professionals. Each chart went through several iterations before it assumed its current form. The development process used to design the charts should, therefore, ensure a high degree of content validity (i.e., the degree to which each chart adequately captures the entire attribute it is intended to measure).

Methods of Administration

The COOP charts were designed to fit into the standard data collection routine of busy ambulatory practices. The charts can be administered via two modes: (i) clinician administered (physician, nurse, medical assistant) or (ii) patient self-administered.

The first method requires the assistance of a nurse, medical assistant, or whoever is responsible for measuring vital signs, height, weight, and blood pressure. The patient is shown the charts one at a time and is asked to read the question carefully and to indicate the answer that best depicts his/her status. Answers or scores are recorded in the patient's medical record, on a flow sheet, or in the progress note for that visit.

The second method utilizes the time spent by the patient in the waiting area of the practitioner's office. A patient, upon reporting to the receptionist, is handed a standard packet of charts and an answer sheet. The patient is instructed to read the charts and circle the score (i.e., 1 to 5 for each chart listed on the answer sheet that best depicts his/her status). Most patients can complete all nine charts in less than five minutes. The answer sheet is placed in the patient's medical record and forwarded to the clinician. Charts may be used selectively and each requires about 30 to 45 seconds to complete.

Methods for Evaluating the COOP Chart System

This chapter explains how the COOP charts were evaluated through their use on over 1,400 patients sampled from four clinical settings. Each setting used different protocols to evaluate one or more aspects of the charts. Results from each setting were handled and analyzed independently. Profiles of the study settings are shown in Table 8.2.

The methods used to asses the variability, reliability, validity, acceptability, and clinical utility of the COOP charts are summarized next.

Variability

A comprehensive analysis of both single-item and multiitem measures demands rigorous testing with diverse populations. A useful instrument must be sensitive enough to detect differences between patients (i.e., to show variability). Because of the nature of single-item instruments, the principle of variability becomes very important.

Reliability

The initial and perhaps the most important question asked by clinicians about any measurement instrument is how dependable is it? A clinician, through daily medical use, develops a certain degree of trust in his/her instruments (i.e., blood pressure cuff, stethoscope, thermometer). Thus high reliability is an essential feature of any useful tool. Although some error is inevitable in any measurement instrument, a perfectly reliable tool will reflect only those changes in measurement values that are true differences (i.e., not changes in values due to random error). We used two conventional methods to assess the reliability of the charts. It should be noted that the internal consistency approach to reliability assessment is not applicable to the charts because they are single-item measures.

TEST–RETEST RELIABILITY

This form of reliability involves the assessment of an individual patient at two points in time by the same method of administration and then a comparison of the results. Several test–retest studies were done. In two settings (i.e., the VA and Bowman Gray), patients were assessed with the charts by the same research assistant twice, with an interval of about one hour between each assessment. In Bowman Gray, patients were also assessed (usually by telephone with a take-home copy of the charts available), approximately 2 weeks later (average, 16 days). This time interval was varied to determine the

TABLE 8.2. Clinical settings in which COOP charts were evaluated.

Place[a]	Setting	Patients	Evaluation purpose
COOP (1)	Small private practices in rural New England	Adults visiting office practices, predominantly white, with common acute and chronic diseases, 57% female, average age 60 $N = 372$	Different examiner reliability Validity Acceptability Clinical utility
VA (2)	VA Outpatient Department in rural area	Elderly males, predominantly white, lower income, under care for chronic problems, 0% female, average age 70 $N = 231$	Validity Test–retest reliability (1 hour)
BG (3)	Free clinic & university outpatient department in urban area	Low-income hypertensive and diabetic patients, 46% black, 66% female, average age 59 $N = 51$	Test–retest reliability (1 hour and 2 weeks)
MOS (4)	Primary care and specialty solo and group practices in urban areas	Diabetic, cardiac, hypertensive and depressed patients under care in different systems of health care, 57% female, average age 58 $N = 784$	Validity

[a] (1) COOP Primary Care Practices — included predominantly small-town, middle-to upper-income patients visiting their primary care physician; (2) Veterans Administration Outpatient Clinic, WRJ — included rural male veterans age 65 and older; (3) Bowman Gray School of Medicine — included predominantly urban, lower-income patients visiting either a hypertension or diabetes clinic; (4) Medical Outcomes Study — included chronic disease patients in three urban areas (Chicago, Boston, and Los Angeles). Analysis restricted to 784 patients of medical providers who completed charts as part of independent health examinations.

stability of chart scores over time. Because the samples in these two settings were of older and more disadvantaged patients than average, these tests are somewhat stringent. For the use of these measures for decisions regarding individual patients, a reliability of 0.90 or higher has been recommended (13). This standard would be applicable to the Pearson product-moment correlations for the one-hour test–retest results.

TEST–RETEST RELIABILITY WITH DIFFERENT EXAMINERS

This type of reliability measures the extent to which two or more examiners (i.e., people who use the charts to assess patients) obtain scores that agree with one another concerning a given phenomenon at a fixed time interval (i.e., on the same day). In the New London COOP site, the physician and nurse/medical assistant used the charts to obtain scores from the same patients. A trial of test–retest reliability with different examiners was conducted in medical practices under regular field conditions. First, during the period of time when vital signs are measured and a brief history of the presenting problem is taken, the patients ($N = 41$) were assessed with four charts by the office nurse/medical assistant. Second, approximately 20 minutes later, the clinician, blind to the results obtained by the nurse/medical assistant, used the four charts at the conclusion of the clinical encounter. The scores obtained by both methods were compared. The more reliable the charts, the greater the agreement expected between scores.

Two statistics, Pearson's product–moment correlation and Kappa, were used to measure the level of agreement. The Kappa statistic is a more rigorous test of agreement because it corrects for agreement between raters that is due to chance, whereas Pearson's correlation simply reflects the consistency of the rank ordering. Because these two statistics measure two different things— direct agreement versus rank order agreement—it is possible to have high Pearson values and substantially lower Kappa coefficients.

To provide consistency of interpretation, Kappa reliability correlations in the following ranges were given these descriptive labels: "excellent," > .74; "good," .60 to .74; "fair," .40 to .59; and "poor," < .40. These are consistent with guidelines provided by Fleiss (14).

Validity

A second question posed by clinicians of measurement instruments is how accurately does the tool measure what it was designed to measure? For example, a caliper may provide a reliable measure of body fat but it is not a valid measure of body weight. The COOP charts are designed to measure how patients feel and function and how they perceive their health. The charts are valid to the extent that the scores they provide reflect these concepts and not, for example, patients' understanding of functioning as an abstract term. The empirical validity of the COOP charts has been evaluated using several approaches.

ASSOCIATION WITH VALIDITY INDICATOR VARIABLES

One common way to assess validity is to determine the degree of correlation between a new measure and other factors (i.e., validity indicator variables) that should in theory be related to the new measure. We assessed this type of empirical validity by testing the relationship between the charts and selected demographic variables and health measures. In general, we expected that higher levels of dysfunction as measured with the charts would be directly associated with worse levels of health status, using other indicators of health. The following measures were used as health-related validity indicator variables: number of disability days; number of symptoms; level of cognitive function; number of sleep disturbances and sleep respiratory problems; reported walking pace; energy/fatigue level; perceived resistance to illness; health outlook and health distress; and satisfaction with family, family function, and reported life events.

CONVERGENT VALIDITY: ASSOCIATION WITH PAIRED MEASURES

Another common method for evaluating empirical validity is to measure the degree of association between a new measure and a previously validated measure that theoretically reflects a similar phenomenon of interest. For example, many of the charts were designed to measure areas similar but not identical to the Medical Outcome Study (MOS) "long-form" measures cited earlier in the text (Table 8.2). The paired chart and long-form relationships we were able to evaluate are shown in Table 8.3.

If the charts have convergent validity, then one would expect to observe moderate to strong correlations between each respective chart and the relevant paired measure. It was expected that the new chart measures would be significantly related to existing multiitem measures and that most correlations would be in the range of 0.50 to 0.75 (i.e., similar to correlations that other health status instruments have shown when compared to one another).

TABLE 8.3. COOP Charts and MOS paired measures.

Chart	Paired measure
Physical	Physical functioning: $k = 10$
Emotional	Emotional status: $32, k = 32$
Daily work	Role limitations: $k = 13$
Social	Social role limitations: $k = 4$
Pain	Pain: $k = 12$
Overall condition	Current health: $k = 7$
Social support	Social support: $k = 19$

DISCRIMINANT VALIDITY: MULTITRAIT–MULTIMETHOD ANALYSIS

A particularly powerful way to evaluate discriminant validity (in addition to convergent validity) is to use a technique known as multitrait–multimethod (MTMM) analysis (15, 16). In the MTMM approach, one set of measures (i.e., the charts) and a corresponding set of measures that is constructed differently (i.e., the relevant multiitem measures that correspond to the charts) are compared to assess "convergent" and "discriminant" validity. If discriminant validity is good, then correlations between different measures of the same concept (e.g., COOP physical and long-form physical) should exceed correlations among different concepts measured either by different methods—heteromethod correlations (e.g., COOP physical with long-form mental) or by the same method—monomethod correlations (e.g., COOP physical with COOP mental). The Hays–Hayashi MTMM quality index, which ranges from negative infinity to +1.0, provides an overall indication of the convergent and discriminant validity.

KNOWN-GROUPS VALIDITY

To establish known-groups validity, the scores of one known group on some variable of interest are compared to the scores of another known group on that same variable of interest. The term *known groups* is based on the knowledge of group membership on one factor that is normally associated with a certain level for the variable of interest. For example, a new measure of socioeconomic status should produce higher values for a group of "documented" wealthy individuals than for a group of "documented" indigent individuals.

We used a known-group approach to determine if the COOP charts were as accurate as the MOS short-form survey (17) at "detecting" the impact of disease on patient functioning. This was done by using 20 measures of disease status and demographic variables as independent variables (i.e., known diagnostic and socioeconomic groups) and treating the COOP chart and MOS short-form measures, respectively, as dependent variables. Dependent variables were all transformed linearly to a common 0 to 100 score distribution in a multiple regression analysis. If the COOP charts are as valid as the MOS measures, then the independent variables (such as presence or absence of congestive heart failure, arthritis, and depression) should have comparable direct effects on the outcome variable (e.g., physical function measured by the COOP charts versus the MOS measure). The MOS short-form data were gathered on a questionnaire that was completed by patients when they visited their physician, whereas the COOP chart data were collected by trained nurses during a standardized clinical assessment conducted from two to four months later. This lag time between the MOS short-form and the chart data collection points may make the results of the known-groups analysis somewhat more difficult to interpret because both measures were not completed at the same point in time. Consequently, the health status of patients could have changed over the interval, thereby attenuating the effects of disease on the measures of function. This would have the effect of making the charts appear less sensitive to the influence of disease.

Acceptability and Clinical Utility

In an effort to meet the needs of practicing physicians, two additional criteria were used to assess the value of the COOP charts—acceptability and clinical utility.

If the COOP chart system is going to be both useful and used, then it is essential that the main consumers of the system—clinicians and patients—judge them to be acceptable in routine use. Indicators used to assess the acceptability of the charts to practitioners and patients were as follows:

How do the clinicians and patients react to use of the charts? For example, do they enjoy using the charts and view them as easy to understand and answer?

Does the chart system fit into the data collection routine of office practice? For example, can the charts be easily integrated into routine data collection?

A preliminary investigation of the charts on the management of patients was conducted. Full assessment of their utility will be conducted in subsequent studies. Our studies used three indicator variables:

Do the charts affect the communication between the patient and the clinician?

Do the charts provide the clinician with new or useful information about the patient?

Do the charts stimulate new management actions in the care of the patient?

We used two methods to rate the acceptability and clinical utility of the charts. First, patients, nurses, and physicians rated these factors on a questionnaire after the charts had been used on primary care patients visiting 11 office practices in New England. Second, debriefing interviews were conducted with the 11 COOP physicians involved.

The charts were also used by 15 additional physicians located in the United States, Canada, Japan, Holland, Israel, and Australia. These clinicians, although not involved in the major studies listed in Table 8.2, used the charts for periods of time ranging from several weeks to over one year and provided feedback regarding their clinical utility. A total of 23 case histories of patients for whom the charts made a favorable difference in patient care were provided during the debriefing interviews with these 26 clinicians.

Results

This section presents the results of our evaluation of the COOP charts, focusing on their variability, reliability, validity, acceptability, and clinical utility.

Variability

Table 8.4 shows the mean and standard deviation of the nine charts in different patient populations. All the charts had substantial variation in scores: standard deviations ranged from 0.66 to 1.6 and the full range of scores was observed on all charts. Setting aside the health change chart—which requires a different interpretation—the mean scores range from a low of 1.3 (social support in COOP practices) to a high of 3.2 (overall health in VA). Most measures were somewhat skewed towards the good health end of the scale; the measure that was most skewed was social support.

Reliability

Table 8.5 summarizes the test–retest and interrater reliability findings on the COOP charts; r is Pearson's product–moment correlation and K is kappa.

TEST–RETEST AT RELIABILITY WITH THE SAME METHOD OF ADMINISTRATION

The reliability of the COOP charts was outstanding in the one-hour test–retest studies.

In the VA sample, correlation coefficients ranged from 0.93 to 0.99 and Kappa coefficients were all in the excellent range (i.e., from 0.80 to 0.97).

In the Bowman Gray sample, correlation coefficients ranged from 0.74 to 0.98 and five Kappa coefficients were excellent, three were good, and one was fair. As expected, because of the lower socioeconomic status of the Bowman Gray sample, reliability tended to be lower for most of the charts in this population.

These findings suggest that most charts exhibit strong test–retest reliability even when used on elderly and socially disadvantaged patients.

Of course, the relatively short time interval may have resulted in inflated reliability estimates because of recall effects. Consequently, in addition to the one-hour test–retest reliability study, an assessment of the two-week reliability was also conducted at Bowman Gray. The product–moment correlations ranged from 0.42 to 0.88. Physical function had the highest correlation and quality of life the lowest. As expected, reliabilities were lower for most charts at two weeks than at one hour. The lower level of agreement may be due to a change in "actual" health status or to less recall of prior ratings.

TEST–RETEST RELIABILITY WITH DIFFERENT ADMINISTRATORS

The results shown in Table 8.5 on different examiner reliability indicate eight of the nine correlation coefficients were 0.76 or better, whereas role function was 0.60. Four of the charts had excellent Kappa coefficients, two good, and three fair or poor.

TABLE 8.4. Descriptive statistics: Means and standard deviations of chart scores in different patient samples.[a]

COOP chart	COOP[b] Mean (N = 225)	SD	COOP[c] Mean (N = 147)	SD	VA[d] Mean N = 231	SD	BG[e] Mean N = 51	SD	MOS[f] Mean N = 784	SD
Physical function	2.8	1.2	2.6	1.3	2.5	1.3	3.1	1.6	2.4	1.2
Emotional status	2.1	1.1	2.6	1.2	2.1	1.0	2.2	1.2	2.0	1.1
Role function	1.9	1.0	2.2	1.1	2.4	1.3	2.0	1.2	1.7	1.0
Social function	1.8	1.0	1.9	1.1	1.9	1.2	1.8	1.3	1.6	0.9
Pain	2.5	1.3	2.6	1.3	1.5	1.0	2.5	1.5	2.5	1.3
Health change	2.5	.99	2.8	1.0	2.9	0.8	2.7	0.9	3.3	0.8
Overall health	2.8	1.0	3.0	1.0	3.2	0.9	2.9	1.2	2.6	1.0
Social support	1.3	.66	1.9	1.1	1.6	1.2	1.9	1.4	1.7	1.1
Quality of life	1.8	.87	2.2	0.9	—[g]	—[g]	2.2	1.0	2.1	0.8

[a] Chart scores range from 1 to 5; 5 indicates poorest health except for Health Change Chart scores for which a score of 3 indicates "no change"; 1 and 2 indicate improvement; and 4 and 5 indicate decline in health.
[b] New London Medical Center COOP Practices.
[c] General COOP Practices.
[d] Veterans Administration Outpatient clinic, WRJ.
[e] Bowman Gray School of Medicine.
[f] Medical Outcomes study.
[g] The Chart was not used in this sample.

TABLE 8.5. Reliability of COOP charts: test–retest reliability in different patient samples.

	Patient sample							
	VA Test–retest 1 Hr		Bowman Gray Test–retest 1 Hr		Bowman Gray[a] Test–retest 2 Wks		New London Test–retest RN & MD	
COOP chart	r	k	r	k	r	k	r	k
Physical function	.96	.85	.98	.87	.83	.51	.76	.37
Emotional status	.96	.80	.79	.55	.66	.49	.92	.81
Role function	.98	.95	.87	.68	.88	.63	.60	.56
Social function	.99	.94	.94	.79	.64	.42	.87	.63
Pain	.96	.87	.98	.90	.74	.52	.98	.87
Health change	.99	.97	.87	.76	NR[b]	NR[b]	.79	.58
Overall health	.98	.94	.89	.67	.71	.53	.81	.63
Social support	.93	.86	.91	.76	.46	.32	.81	.79
Quality of life	NA[c]	NA[c]	.74	.65	.42	.29	.88	.69
Number in sample	53[d]		51		51		41	

[a] These Bowman Gray patients cited above were given the COOP Charts again approximately two weeks post base line; the average interval was 16 days.
[b] NR indicates that this value is not relevant. This is because the Health Change Chart is designed to monitor relatively minor fluctuations in health over time. The correlation coefficient for test–retest at two weeks was .25.
[c] NA denotes this correlation was not ascertained because the chart was not given.
[d] Numbers in the VA and the COOP (New London) sample do not equal the total number of patients listed in Table 8.2 because these reliability studies were conducted on a subsample of patients.

TABLE 8.6. Validity correlations between COOP charts and selected MOS measures ($N = 784$).

Validity Measure	COOP Chart[a]							
	Physical function	Emotional status	Role function	Social function	Pain	Overall health	Social resources	Quality of life
Disability days	.14[b]	.10[b]	.25[b]	.15[b]	.14[b]	.20[b]	.04	.16[b]
Symptoms	.31[b]	.40[b]	.48[b]	.42[b]	.53[b]	.53[b]	.24[b]	.39[b]
Cognitive function	.12[b]	.52[b]	.35[b]	.48[b]	.21[b]	.43[b]	.32[b]	.41[b]
Sleep problems	.21[b]	.44[b]	.41[b]	.44[b]	.36[b]	.51[b]	.31[b]	.41[b]
Walking pace	.30[b]	.02	.24[b]	.16[b]	.15[b]	.16[b]	.04	.16[b]
Energy/Fatigue	.37[b]	.40[b]	.53[b]	.44[b]	.39[b]	.58[b]	.22[b]	.38[b]
Resistance to illness	.18[b]	.23[b]	.28[b]	.24[b]	.27[b]	.39[b]	.19[b]	.27[b]
Health outlook	.26[b]	.19[b]	.27[b]	.26[b]	.24[b]	.39[b]	.15[b]	.26[b]
Health distress	.29[b]	.41[b]	.47[b]	.51[b]	.36[b]	.52[b]	.26[b]	.38[b]
Family satisfaction	.00	.39[b]	.18[b]	.28	.13[b]	.29[b]	.39[b]	.41[b]
Family functioning	.04	.37[b]	.16[b]	.23[b]	.16[b]	.23[b]	.39[b]	.40[b]
Life events	.06	.38[b]	.22[b]	.27	.16[b]	.20[b]	.18[b]	.34[b]

[a] All measures are scored so that a higher score indicates poorer health, fewer resources, or poorer quality of life.
[b] $p < .05$.

Validity

Tables 8.6 to 8.11 show the empirical validity of the charts.

ASSOCIATION WITH VALIDITY INDICATOR VARIABLES

Table 8.6 presents correlations between COOP charts and established measures of health, perceptions of health, and other validity indicator variables for 784 chronic disease patients. These variables were selected to represent the range of possible health and related measures from the MOS base-line patient assessment questionnaire.

The results show that, almost without exception, the association between the charts and the validity variables is statistically significant in the expected direction. More subjective health measures—for example, symptoms, energy/fatigue, resistance to illness, health outlook, and health distress—tend to correlate somewhat more highly with the charts than do the more objective measures such as disability days and walking pace.

Life events, family functioning, and family satisfaction have significant effects on all charts except physical function. Social support was least related to other health measures; this is as expected because it is the most removed from health.

The empirical validity of the COOP charts was further explored by examining their correlations with selected clinical measures in the VA sample. Table 8.7 reveals moderate correlations in the expected direction between chart scores and clinical measures. For example, the correlations of number of symptoms with chart scores range from 0.25 (health change) to 0.51 (overall health) and were all statistically significant. The chronic illness score was significantly associated with all the charts except emotional status and health

TABLE 8.7. Validity correlations between the COOP charts[a] and selected clinical measures in the VA sample[b] ($N = 231$).

| COOP chart | Clinical measure[b] | | |
	Symptom score	Chronic illness score	Number of medicines
Physical function	.36[c]	.22[c]	.18[c]
Emotional status	.46[c]	.10	.16[c]
Role function	.45[c]	.32[c]	.42[c]
Social function	.48[c]	.26[c]	.32[c]
Pain	.34[c]	.34[c]	.32[c]
Health change	.25[c]	.11	.08
Overall health	.51[c]	.23[c]	.23[c]
Social support	.27[c]	.16[c]	.06

[a]The Quality of Life Chart is not included because it had not been developed when these data were collected.
[b]Clinical measures included "symptom score," which was based on the frequency (never, seldom, sometimes, often, always) of 36 symptoms reported by patients over a one-month interval. The chronic illness score was based on a review of patients' medical records and scored according to the system developed by Linn and Gurel (18). Number of medicines was based on a review of patients' medical charts and represents the number of prescribed medications currently taken by the patient at least three times per week or more.
[c]$p < .05$.

change. The number of medications was significantly related to all charts except health change and social support.

CONVERGENT VALIDITY

As discussed above, one way to establish the validity of a new measure is to determine how well it correlates with previously validated measures. Table 8.8 shows correlations between the charts and paired MOS measures of health in three different samples (VA, COOP: New London, and MOS).

On the whole, the correlations between the charts and the paired measures were impressive. The correlations ranged from 0.48 to 0.78 with the majority in the 0.60 to 0.70 range. In addition, shared variance between charts and paired measures was substantial, ranging from 20 to 61% for physical function, 38 to 49% for emotional function, 35 to 42% for role function, and 26 to 35% for

TABLE 8.8. Convergent validity: correlations between COOP charts and MOS long-form measures in different patient samples.

COOP chart and paired RAND measure[a]	Site[b]		
	Veterans Administration	New London	MOS
Physical function chart			
Physical function (K = 10)	–	.78 (N = 99)	.59 (N = 703)
Physical function (K = 11)	.68 (N = 231)	–	–
Emotional status chart			
MHI (K = 5)	.70 (N = 231)	.67 (N = 77)	.64 (N = 717)
MHI (K = 17)	–	–	.67 (N = 718)
MHI (K = 32)	–	–	.68 (N = 719)
MHI (K = 46)	.62 (N = 80)	–	–
Role function chart			
Role functioning (K = 2)	.65 (N = 231)	–	–
Role functioning (K = 6)	–	.62 (N = 100)	–
Role functioning (K = 13)	–	–	.59 (N = 701)
Social function chart			
Social activities (K = 2)	–	.54 (N = 76)	–
Social activities (K = 4)	–	–	.61 (N = 704)
Pain chart			
Pain rating (K = 1)	–	.74 (N = 76)	.63 (N = 695)
Pain (K = 12)	–	–	.61 (N = 700)
Overall health chart			
Current health (K = 4)	.51 (N = 231)	.56 (N = 68)	–
Current health (K = 6)	–	–	.61 (N = 707)
Social support chart			
Social support (K = 5)	–	.61 (N = 67)	–
Social support (K = 9)	.65 (N = 231)	–	–
Social support (K = 19)	–	–	.48 (N = 664)

[a] The rows show the names of seven COOP Charts and the paired MOS measures. The number of items in each paired MOS measure (K) is shown in parentheses. The number of items varies at times from those cited earlier in the text because preliminary versions of the MOS measures were used in earlier studies.
[b] The columns show results on the convergent validity using Pearson's correlation coefficients to measure the association between seven COOP Charts (physical, emotional, role, social function, pain, overall health, and social support) and relevant paired MOS measures. The size of the sample (N) is shown in parentheses.

overall health. These relations suggest that the charts tap information similar to that measured by longer, standardized health measures and provide support for the convergent validity of the charts.

DISCRIMINANT VALIDITY: MULTITRAIT–MULTIMETHOD ANALYSIS

Table 8.9 displays the results of an MTMM analysis conducted on 592 chronic disease patients with complete data on these variables. The average convergent validity correlation (i.e., correlation between corresponding chart and MOS measures) was 0.60, whereas the average off-diagonal correlation was 0.16, which is considerably smaller than the average validity correlation. This provides general support for the discriminant validity of the measures.

To assess discriminant validity in further detail, we compared convergent validity correlation with appropriate off-diagonal correlations following the Campbell and Fiske (15) 1959 guidelines. Different measures of the same trait tended to correlate significantly more highly with one another than did measures of different traits (i.e., 96% of the heteromethod and 70% of the monomethod comparisons were statistically significant in the hypothesized direction). The Hays–Hayashi: Quality Index was 0.82, which indicates generally good discriminant validity for the measures.

Although the convergent and discriminant validity of most charts were quite good, there were two trouble spots. Role and social function had clear discriminant validity problems: only 50% and 42%, respectively, of monomethod comparisons were statistically significant in the hypothesized direction.

Similar findings to those just cited above were obtained from the MTMM analysis performed on 229 elderly patients in the VA sample (see Table 8.10).

KNOWN GROUPS

The results shown in Table 8.11 provide convincing and striking evidence to support the validity of the COOP charts. These results show that the COOP charts are indeed sensitive to the effects of disease. That is to say, the presence of medically verified diseases has a measurable influence—in the expected way—on the level of patients' health as measured by the charts. Table 8.11 presents results on four of the COOP charts; similar findings observed for the other charts are not presented here.

Care must be taken in comparing the parameter estimates related to the charts with those related to the MOS measures because of differences in the standard deviations of the two respective scales and because of the different times the measures were administered. Bearing this in mind, we see that the effects observed for the charts mirror, for the most part, those observed for the MOS short-form health measures. Except for emotional status, the amount of explained variance was similar in the corresponding chart and MOS measures. For example, the proportion of variance explained for the chart and MOS physical function measures were 30% and 27%, respectively. In addition

TABLE 8.9. MTMM matrix from MOS sample ($N = 592$).

Functional measures	COOP charts							RAND scales						
	Physical function	Emotional status	Role function	Social function	Pain	Overall health	Social support	Physical function	Emotional function	Role function	Social function	Pain	Overall health	Social support
COOP charts														
Physical function	1.00													
Emotional status	.02	1.00												
Role function	.37	.35	1.00											
Social function	.25	.52	.56	1.00										
Pain	.28	.26	.47	.34	1.00									
Overall health	.39	.46	.53	.46	.43	1.00								
Social support	.13	.35	.19	.27	.19	.32	1.00							
RAND scales														
Physical function	.60[a]	.11	.52	.38	.40	.47	.15	1.00						
Emotional status	.02	.66[a]	.33	.49	.26	.44	.47	.19	1.00					
Role function	.43	.26	.58[a]	.46	.38	.53	.22	.67	.40	1.00				
Social function	.29	.37	.49	.58[a]	.33	.50	.23	.52	.58	.62	1.00			
Pain	.35	.33	.55	.42	.63[a]	.52	.23	.62	.39	.65	.57	1.00		
Overall health	.42	.33	.49	.43	.45	.63[a]	.28	.64	.42	.63	.58	.60	1.00	
Social support	.06	.37	.20	.26	.17	.27	.50[a]	.15	.50	.23	.23	.18	.20	1.00

[a] Convergent correlations. The average convergent validity equals 0.60; the average off-diagonal correlations is 0.16; the Hays-Hayashi MTMM Quality Index equals 0.82.

TABLE 8.10. MTMM matrix from the VA sample of elderly patients ($N = 229$).

Functional measures	COOP charts[a]					RAND scales				
	Physical function	Emotional status	Role function	Overall health	Social support	Physical function	Emotional status	Role function	Overall health	Social support
COOP charts										
Physical function	1.00									
Emotional status	.18	1.00								
Role function	.59	.33	1.00							
Overall health	.37	.32	.48	1.00						
Social support	.09	.19	.20	.13	1.00					
RAND scales										
Physical function	.68[a]	.30	.71	.47	.16	1.00				
Emotional status	.13	.70[a]	.28	.32	.23	.25	1.00			
Role function	.51	.32	.64[a]	.40	.16	.68	.24	1.00		
Overall health	.32	.42	.58	.53[a]	.24	.48	.50	.49	1.00	
Social support	.00	.23	.11	.04	.65[a]	.15	.30	.16	.19	1.00

[a]Convergent correlations. The average convergent validity equals 0.64; average off-diagonal correlations is 0.32; Hays-Hayashi MTMM Quality Index equals 0.83.

TABLE 8.11. Comparison of COOP charts with paired RAND measures: proportion of variance in COOP chart scores and RAND measure scores explained by diagnostic status and demographic characteristics.[a]

Variables in Regression[b]	Physical function (N = 603)		Emotional status (N = 631)		Role function (N = 592)		Overall health (N = 1865)	
	COOP charts	MOS	COOP charts	MOS	COOP charts	MOS	COOP charts	MOS
Diagnostic Status[c]								
Diabetes	-4.74	-10.69[a]	-0.55	-1.53	-2.52	1.18	-6.16[a]	-11.34[a]
Myocardial infarction	-27.09[a]	-32.70[a]	3.17	0.24	-11.40[a]	-46.61[a]	-8.89	-13.58[a]
Congestive Heart Failure	-18.30[a]	-30.68[a]	7.45	0.05	-20.49[a]	-44.53[a]	-11.42[a]	-26.36[a]
Hypertension	-7.58[a]	-3.12	0.37	-1.62	-2.21	-3.82	-8.47[a]	-6.01[a]
Arthritis	-2.03	-8.29[a]	-5.21[a]	0.26	-4.76[a]	-12.10[a]	-3.99[a]	-3.00
Lung	-9.45[a]	-17.98[a]	-4.55	-3.52	-5.80	-9.07	-8.62[a]	-14.70[a]
Back	-1.79	1.26	2.98	3.34	0.84	7.07	-3.81	-5.82
Gastrointestinal	-9.10[a]	-2.60	-6.77	-3.39	-12.67[a]	-13.54[a]	-13.38[a]	-10.85[a]
Angina	-13.10[a]	-21.95[a]	-5.25	-2.79	-9.65[a]	-10.84[a]	-5.99	-11.49[a]
Depressive symptoms	-3.68	-10.44[a]	-26.24[a]	-29.39[a]	-13.84[a]	-15.05[a]	-18.28[a]	-15.14[a]
Diagnostic problem	0.07	2.14	-4.10	-2.21	4.13	10.71	-5.19	-2.28
Amputation	3.07	16.57[a]	-2.62	11.17[a]	8.13	15.20	3.25	16.61[a]

Other major problems	−10.86[a]	−10.65[a]	−4.12	−2.68	−11.40[a]	−15.43[a]	−11.24[a]	−8.59[a]
Heart failure	7.46	3.02	−11.03[a]	−5.16	−8.28	−18.33[a]	−8.14	−13.16[a]
Kidney Disease	−24.66[a]	−12.80	−1.46	−6.10	−8.28	−16.47	−10.56	−23.25[a]
Trouble seeing	0.83	−2.69	−1.48	−1.62	−2.05	−3.54	−5.20	−5.54
Demographic Status								
Gender (male)	16.41[a]	6.10[a]	7.13[a]	0.55	6.56[a]	6.72[a]	4.35[a]	2.01
Age	−0.39[a]	−0.08	0.19[a]	0.22[a]	0.05	−0.01	0.12	0.08
Education	1.05[a]	−0.09	−0.10	−0.04	−0.06	0.43	0.37	0.33
Income	0.03	0.14	0.01	0.05	−0.04	0.11	0.04	0.20[a]
Intercept	79.74	88.65	82.74	84.07	93.22	91.00	78.26	74.21
R-square[d]	0.30	0.27	0.29	0.52	0.23	0.26	0.26	0.35

[a] $p < .05$.
[b] A multivariate analysis was conducted using the COOP chart or RAND measure score as the dependent variable and 21 clinical and demographic variables as independent variables. Results for the most important variables are shown. The values listed for each independent variable are unstandardized beta weights. An example of how to interpret the beta weight follows. Starting with the intercept value of 79.74 (column 1) the effect of having a myocardial infarction (the second diagnostic variable) is to reduce the predicted score on physical function (as measured by the COOP chart) by −27.09 points.
[c] The diagnostic status of each patient was based on information provided by the physician on a special encounter form used for research except for "arthritis" and "depression symptoms," which were based on data provided by the patient.
[d] The R-square value represents the proportion of variance in the dependent variable explained by the independent variables included in the regression model.

to similarities in the proportion of variance explained, the predictor variables used for both the chart and MOS regressions tend to (i) have the same sign [i.e., the effect of having a diagnosed myocardial infarction (MI) is to decrease the predicted health score registered by both the chart and MOS measures on physical, role, and overall health] and (ii) similar patterns of statistical significance (i.e., the effect of MI significantly decreases the predicted score for physical, role, and overall health measures).

The emotional function difference in proportion of variance explained was substantial: r^2 for the chart versus the MOS measure were 0.30 and 0.52, respectively. This difference was largely attributable to the level of correlation between depressive symptoms and emotional status as defined by the charts and the MOS measures ($r = 0.49$ versus 0.69; standardized betas $= -0.41$ versus -0.64).

Acceptability

In addition to reliability and validity, the charts were also evaluated for acceptability to patients and clinicians. Post-visit questionnaires completed by 5 office nurses and 225 patients, respectively, showed that 89% of the patients enjoyed the charts and 93% of the patients reported that they liked the chart illustrations. Nurse-rated enjoyment of the charts by patients and patients' liking of the illustrations did not differ significantly by patients' sex, age, educational level, or marital status.

According to the nurses, 99% of the patients understood the charts, whereas 97% of the patients reported understanding them. Understanding of charts did not differ by demographic variables.

Debriefing interviews with office staff from 10 practices indicated that (i) the charts are not difficult to integrate into the practice's routine for gathering information on patients and (ii) a four-chart set took two to three minutes for nurses to use with patients.

Clinical Utility

Highlights of the debriefing interviews are provided in 21 case histories, which are included in Appendix B. This qualitative information showed that use of the charts

Regularly provided important information for both new and established patients;

frequently led to the discovery of previously unrecognized problems that often revealed greater dysfunction than had previously been recognized;

at times showed the patient to be functioning better than expected, given the disease status; and

improved communication between patients and clinicians.

In addition, we learned that some clinicians seemed to attribute more value to the charts than other clinicians. For example, physicians' ratings of chart utility differed significantly across individuals.

The effect of the charts on physician–patient communication (as viewed by the physician) was rated as positive for 13% of the patients, no effect for 85% of the patients, and negative for 2% of the patients.

An important finding was that physician-completed, post-visit questionnaires showed that for 25% of patients seen, the charts led to new information. Moreover, physicians reported that this new information led to changes in their clinical management in 40% of patients in which this new information was uncovered. This suggests that use of the charts may stimulate changes in what physicians know about their patients and how they treat their patients, which, in theory, could lead to subsequent improvements in health status.

PATIENT'S VIEW OF CLINICAL UTILITY

Patient post-visit questionnaire results provide further evidence of the utility of the charts. For example, almost 9 out of 10 of the COOP primary care patients reported that the information provided by the charts was important for their doctor to know. More than 75% of the patients indicated that the charts influenced their communication with the doctor; 85% indicated that the charts affected management actions. Most patients rated the charts as useful: 10%, excellent; 21%, very good; 43%, good; 23%, fair; and 3%, poor. Patient ratings of utility were unrelated to more demographic variables. However, the effect of the charts on communication was related to the sex of patients such that 86% of the males versus 69% of the females reported that the charts influenced their communication with the physician.

Discussion

In this section we (i) summarize our results and discuss their implications for clinical practice, (ii) relate our findings to some of the relevant literature, and (iii) cite the limitations of the work performed to date and discuss possible directions for the future.

Results Summary and Implications for Clinical Practice

We set out to develop a set of measures that could be used in busy office practices to screen and monitor patient functioning. What did we learn on the positive side? First, we found that the charts are reliable. They generate reproducible results when used properly with patients. Although the reliability of self-administration was not tested, it would probably yield similar results. Second, we found that the charts produce valid information. The charts are strongly associated with related measures that have undergone validation, they are correlated with health and clinical status in the expected manner, and perhaps most importantly, they detect dysfunction associated with major chronic diseases. Third, we learned that the "consumers" involved in the measurement of patient function—physicians, office nurses, and patients—all indicated that the charts could be beneficial and were not difficult to use, understand, or interpret. Most patients enjoyed using the charts and believed that they measured important aspects of health. Fourth, with respect to clinical utility, physicians who used the charts indicated that they generated new information on about one out of four patients. The more than 20 clinical case studies we collected provided further evidence to support the clinical utility of the charts.

What did we learn on the negative side? First, we learned that there are occasions when the charts may have a deleterious effect on physician–patient communication. This is a very infrequent event–it occurs roughly 2% of the time according to physicians—but it still merits further thought and a note of caution. Second, we found that some of the charts could probably be improved. The MTMM results, although they mostly showed good convergent and discriminant validity, suggest that some of the measures might be further enhanced. For example, there appears to be a good deal of overlap between the COOP chart measures of physical function and role function and the MOS short-form measures of these same functions. Third, we observed that some physicians seemed to attribute more value to the charts than other physicians. For example, physicians' ratings of chart utility differed significantly across individuals. Fourth, we were constantly reminded that even though the charts did not take a long time to fill out, if they were administered by the nurse/medical assistant or the physician, instead of self-administered, there would always be a substantial cost-effectiveness issue. Consequently, we need to determine which charts are most useful for what kinds of patients at what interval of time.

Relationship of COOP Charts to Literature and Other Measures of Function

The methods we used to evaluate the reliability and validity of the charts are generally similar to those that other researchers have used to assess their health status measures. For example, the techniques we used to check reliability and validity are similar to those used to evaluate the RAND health status measures (19), the SIP (8), and the Duke–UNC Health Profile (9). In a very rough way, therefore, it is possible to compare the reliability and validity of the charts with these other multidimensional measures. When this is done, we see that the reliability and validity coefficients of the charts are about the same as those observed for these other measures. For example, the average construct validity correlation for the charts with "paired" measures was approximately 0.60 (e.g., charts versus MOS long-form measures in the MOS sample), whereas the comparable figure for the Duke–UNC Health Profile was 0.49 (e.g., Duke versus SIP).

Perhaps the most impressive findings were obtained from the known diagnostic groups analysis. The empirical validity of the charts was tested in a rigorous, head-to-head match against the MOS short-form measures. The charts were found to do almost as well as these excellent multiitem measures on ability to detect the impact of disease on patient function. This analysis showed that the charts, when compared to the MOS short-form measures, had a similar sensitivity to pick up the effects of disease. It has been demonstrated elsewhere that disease has multiple effects that "ripple out" and consequently affect various dimensions of a person's functioning and well-being. Thus, a vital test of the empirical validity of a functional measure concerns whether it is sensitive to the clinical effects of documented disease. The fact that the charts appear to score as well on reliability, validity, and disease sensitivity as on established, multidimensional measures is noteworthy. This is because the charts use a single, global item to measure what other systems assess with 5 to 40 items or more.

Limitations and Future Directions

Much work has been done to assess the reliability, validity, acceptability, and clinical utility of the chart, but further work is needed. Concerning reliability, it would be useful to expand on the work reported thus far by (i) better determining how reliability varies as a function of clinician, patient, and setting; (ii) conducting more refined reliability studies involving various test–retest time periods and thereby clarifying the importance of the recall factor; and (iii) establishing the reliability of self-administration vis-à-vis clinician administration. With respect to validity, we need to learn more about the ability of the charts to detect actual changes occurring within the individual patient's level of function that take place over time and that are linked to known changes in treatment or natural history. We need to attempt to (i) obtain better discrimination between different dimensions of health and thereby improve our ability to differentiate role function from physical function; (ii) learn how to calibrate the levels of chart scores to clinically relevant events, such as the effect of having an MI or depression; and (iii) determine how to assign weighted values to each of the five levels of each respective chart because the size of the intervals between the levels has not been established even though the rank order is clear. Finally, although the acceptability of the charts was shown to be good in many diverse settings, we know little about (i) how much the charts' illustrations enhance (or detract from) their acceptability and measurement properties or (ii) how easy it would be to disseminate the charts more widely to scores of medical practices across the country.

The ultimate test of the charts' value, however, has to do with their clinical utility. We need to know if regular physicians will really use the charts routinely. If they are used, what new information is produced on what types of patients? How frequently does this new information actually result in a change in the management plan? Finally, how frequently do certain types of patient benefit in terms of measurable gains in function—or less rapid deterioration in function—than would otherwise be the case.

We need to determine if the charts need to be linked, as we think they do, to more in-depth, yet practical assessment tools that physicians can use to work up problem patients. We need to learn whether physicians would benefit from education and training in topics such as a functional approach to patient care and how to evaluate and manage patient function.

Although much work lies ahead, the charts appear to be reliable, valid, and acceptable. Of course, further improvements are needed for the charts to be suitable for use in primary care practice in different parts of the world, but their use with certain types of patients could make an important contribution to better documentation of the outcomes of care. To improve the quality of patient care, we first must have practical means to measure, over time, patients' reasons for their visits, their diagnoses, their treatments, and their treatment outcomes.

Acknowledgment. This work was supported by the Henry J. Kaiser Family Foundation Grant Number 85-3180.

References

1. Nelson EC, Wasson JH, Kirk JW: Assessment of function in routine clinical practice: description of the COOP Chart method and preliminary findings. *J. Chron Dis.* 40(S1):55S, 1987.
2. McDowell I, Newell C: *Measuring Health: A Guide to Rating Scales and Questionnaires.* New York, Oxford University Press, 1987.
3. Katz S, Ford AB, Moskowitz RW, et al.: Studies of illness in the aged. The index of ADL: A standardized measure of biological and psychosocial function. *JAMA.* 185:914, 1963.
4. The Criteria Committee of the New York Heart Association, Inc.: *Diseases of the Heart and Blood Vessels:Nomenclature and Criteria for Diagnosis.* 6th ed. Boston, Little Brown; 1964.
5. Goldman L, Hashimoto B, Cook EF, et al.: Comparative reproducibility and validity of systems for assessing cardiovascular functional class: Advantages of a new specific activity scale. *Circulation.* 64(6):1277, 1981.
6. Nelson E, Conger B, Douglass R, et al.: Functional health status levels of primary care patients. *JAMA.* 249(24):3331–3338, 1983.
7. Ware JE, Johnston SA, Davies-Avery A, et al.: *Conceptualization and measurement of Health for Adults in the Health Insurance Study: Vol III Mental Health.* R-1987/3-HEW. Santa Monica, CA: The Rand Corp., 1979.
8. Bergner M, Bobbitt RA, Carter WB, et al.: The sickness impact profile: Conceptual formulation and methodology for the development of a health status measure. *Int J Health Serv.* 6:393, 1976.

9. Parkerson GR, Gehlbach SH, Wagner EH, et al.: The Duke–UNC health profile: An adult health status instrument for primary care. *Med Care.* 19:806, 1981.

10. Sackett D, Chambers L, MacPherson AS, et al.: The development and application of indices of health: General methods and a summary of results. *American J Public Health.* 67:423–427, 1977.

11. Hunt SM, McEwen J, McKenna SP: Measuring health status: A tool for clinicians and epidemiologists. *JR Coll Gen Pract.* 35:185, 1985.

12. Ware JE Jr.: Standards for validating health measures: Definition and content. *J. Chron Dis.* 40:473–480, 1987.

13. Nunnally C: *Psychometric Theory*, New York, McGraw-Hill, 1978.

14. Powers SA: A PASCAL program to assess the interrater reliability of nominal scales. *Edu Psychol Meas.* 45:613–614, 1985.

15. Campbell DT, Fiske DW: Convergent and discriminant validation by the multitrait-y matrix. *Psychol Bull.* 56:81–105, 1959.

16. Hayashi T, Hays RD. A microcomputer program for analyzing multitrait–multimethod matrices. *Behav Res Methods Instruments and Computer.* 19:345–348,1987. [Also, Santa Monica, CA, The Rand Corp. (P-7298)].

17. Stewart AL, Hays RD, Ware JE: The MOS short-form general health survey: Reliability and validity in a patient population. *Med Care.* 26:724–735, 1988.

18. Linn BF, Gurel L: Cumulative illness rating scale. *JA* Geriatric Society. 16(5):622–626, 1968.

19. Ware JE, Brook RH, Davies-Avery A, et al.: *Conceptualization and Measurement of Health for Adults in the Health Insurance Study: Vol I, Model of Health and Methodology.* Santa Monica, CA, The Rand Corp. (R-1987/1-HEW), 1980.

20. Stewart AL, Greenfield S, Hays RD, et al.: Functional status and well-being of patients with chronic conditions. *JAMA.* 262:907–913, 1989.

Appendix A: Facsimiles of the COOP charts

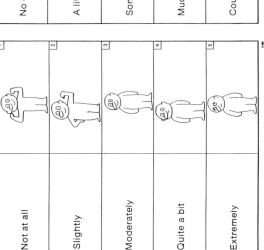

PHYSICAL CONDITION

During the past 4 weeks . . .
What was the most strenuous level
of physical activity you could do for at
least 2 minutes?

Very heavy, e.g.
Run, fast pace
Carry heavy bag of
groceries upstairs

Heavy, e.g.
Jog, slow pace
Climb stairs at moderate
pace

Moderate, e.g.
Walk, fast pace
Garden, easy digging
Carry heavy bag of
groceries

Light, e.g.
Walk, regular pace
Golf or vacuum
Carry light bag of
groceries

Very light, e.g.
Walk, slow pace
Drive car
Wash dishes

EMOTIONAL CONDITION

During the past 4 weeks . . .
How much have you been bothered
by emotional problems such as feeling
unhappy, anxious, depressed, irritable?

Not at all

Slightly

Moderately

Quite a bit

Extremely

DAILY WORK

During the past 4 weeks . . .
How much difficulty did you have doing
your daily work, both inside and outside the
house, because of your physical health or
emotional problems?

No difficulty at all

A little bit of difficulty

Some difficulty

Much difficulty

Could not do

Reprinted with permission.

SOCIAL ACTIVITIES

During the past 4 weeks . . . .
To what extent has your physical health or emotional problems interfered with your normal social activities with family, friends, neighbors or groups?

Not at all	1
Slightly	2
Moderately	3
Quite a bit	4
Extremely	5

4

PAIN

During the past 4 weeks . . . .
How much bodily pain have you generally had?

No pain	1
Very mild pain	2
Mild pain	3
Moderate pain	4
Severe pain	5

5

CHANGE IN CONDITION

How would you rate your physical health and emotional condition now compared to 4 weeks ago?

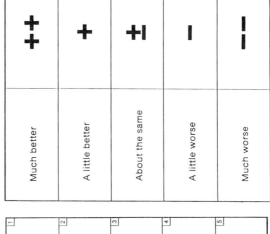

Much better	1
A little better	2
About the same	3
A little worse	4
Much worse	5

6

(continued)

Reprinted with permission.

Appendix A (*Continued*)

OVERALL CONDITION

During the past 4 weeks . . . .
How would you rate your overall
physical health and emotional condition?

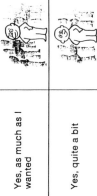

Excellent	1
Very good	2
Good	3
Fair	4
Poor	5

7

SOCIAL SUPPORT

During the past 4 weeks . . . .
Was someone available to help you if you
needed and wanted help? For example if you

— felt very nervous, lonely, or blue
— got sick and had to stay in bed
— needed someone to talk to
— needed help with daily chores
— needed help just taking care of yourself

Yes, as much as I wanted	1
Yes, quite a bit	2
Yes, some	3
Yes, a little	4
No, not at all	5

8

QUALITY OF LIFE

How has the quality of your life been
during the past 4 weeks? i.e. How have
things been going for you?

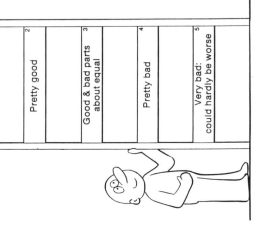

Very well: could hardly be better	1
Pretty good	2
Good & bad parts about equal	3
Pretty bad	4
Very bad: could hardly be worse	5

9

Appendix B: Case Histories on Use of COOP Charts in Primary Care

Introduction

One of the most important ways to document the clinical utility of any functional health assessment tool is to provide actual case histories generated from patients and practitioners using the instrument. Clinicians participating in phase 1 of the COOP study were asked to identify "critical incidents" that highlighted either a positive or negative impact of the charts. A synopsis of 21 different case histories offered by 12 practitioners follow. Clinicians in the Netherlands provided five of the case histories, which demonstrate the potential clinical utility of the charts in other cultures. A summary of the specific clinical benefits of each of the case histories is provided at the conclusion of this section of the report.

Case Histories

Cases histories 1 through 16 were provided from actual clinical encounters between patients and primary care providers in the United States.

Case 1: An established elderly male patient (81 years of age) was under treatment for high blood pressure and arthritis. He was well known by his clinician. During his encounters with the practitioner he complained of fatigue and other nonspecific symptoms. The patient was married and devoted himself to the care of his elderly wife who suffered from Alzheimer's disease. The man received no family support and was not likely to ask for help from others. The clinician characterized the patient as a very gregarious man who created symptoms so he could justify his regular visits to the office. The clinician reported that it was very difficult to accomplish anything with the patient because he denied the root of his problems—he needed respite from the care of his wife. He was invited to participate in the COOP chart study and was given the physical function, role, emotional function, and quality of life charts. The patient scored low on all measures suggesting overall good health. The clinician knew that the patient's only outlet was visits to the office. He confronted the patient about the inconsistencies of his scores. Why was a man who reported a "good" high quality of life and "good" emotional functioning frequenting the office as much as he did? Discussion with the patient revealed that Medicare had refused the man's request for respite because his wife was living in a stable home. The home conditions, however pleasant they were, taxed the patient. The clinician convinced the man to accept help and intervened with Medicare on his behalf.

Case 2: A young man (37 years of age) with no chronic health problems was seen by an emergency physician for an injury to his finger. He saw his clinician a few weeks later for hiatus dysphasia and reported having difficulty swallowing and pain in his finger and arm. He was invited to participate in the study and completed the nine COOP charts. His chart scores were alarming: physical, 4 (poor); emotional, 4 (poor); social function, 3 (moderate); pain, 2 (good); change, 4 (poor); overall health, 4 (poor); social resources, 4 (poor); and quality of life, 3 (poor). The injury had appeared quite trivial to the clinician, but the patient could not function very well, since the pain was located in his dominant hand. The clinician arranged for the man to receive Meals on Wheels. A month later the organic complaint had been relieved without the use of drugs. The man was "significantly better" but still depressed. His depression is being followed. The clinician indicated that the most significant finding of the charts in this instance was the extent of the patient's injury.

Case 3: A 67-year-old man was under treatment for high blood pressure and arthritis. The patient was "vigorous and healthy," according to the clinician. Most of his chart scores (1s or 2s) confirmed this; however, his physical score (3) was much lower than the practitioner had anticipated. It was discovered that the patient had knee trouble and never reported it because he just assumed and accepted that "this was the way it was." He was unaware that something might be done. The clinician and the patient decided to take a more aggressive approach and focus on the arthritic knee condition.

Case 4: A COOP clinician had assumed the care of a 72-year-old patient with chronic obstructive pulmonary disease (COPD) and angina. The patient had suffered a "small" stroke. The patient was given four charts and scored: 5 (poor) on physical; 4 (poor) on role; 3 (moderate) on emotional; and 2 (good) on quality of life. The practitioner was "surprised" and "shocked" that the patient reported being as limited as indicated by his high physical and role chart scores. The clinician aggressively focused on the reason for the patient's low level of functioning and discovered that PVD leg claudication had limited the patient's circulation and was responsible for his dysfunction.

Case 5: A 62-year-old, divorced female was under treatment for palpitations, gastroenteritis, and diarrhea. She was well known to her clinician and had been a regular patient for many years. She was a quiet woman who "kept her chin up" and complained very little. The clinician attributed these traits to the patient's cultural background (Japanese). She was given the charts. Her scores revealed emotional dysfunction (5, poor). The information led the provider to take stronger measures toward treating the patient's emotional health.

Case 6: A 76-year-old male patient was under treatment for high blood pressure, breathing problems, and edema (severe COPD). He was well known to the clinician and had denied the severity of his illness for years. The doctor assumed the patient would score his physical functioning as a 3 (moderate) and was surprised to discover the patient reported a score of 5 (poor). It was the practitioner's first awareness of the patient's limited functional ability. Prior to this point, the clinician was unable to get through the patient's "walls." The short-term management plan will be a stronger, more aggressive treatment without drugs.

Case 7: A 78-year-old male was under treatment for COPD and confusion. According to clinicians who had treated the man's pulmonary condition, he was severely disabled. It was difficult for the clinician to know how much he could "push" the patient due to the patient's "fuzziness" and inconsistency. This resulted in an unclear managment plan. The patient was given the charts. His physical function score was 1 (good). The practitioner was stunned by this and questioned the patient at length. The practitioner had believed that the patient could not function at a high level of activity. In subsequent history taking, the clinician became convinced of the patient's reported functional ability. In this case, the clinician decided he need not develop a more aggressive management plan because the patient's measure of physical performance was satisfactory. The clinician could "back off and not feel guilty." As a result of the charts' scores and increased discussion with the patient, the direction of management became much clearer.

Case 8: An elderly lady was admitted to a local hospital for a cataract operation. She was seen by a COOP clinician for the first time prior to the surgery. She appeared to be in good health. During the exam she indicated that she needed medication to sleep and was bothered by nerves. She did not appear overly anxious or depressed. She was given the COOP charts because the clinician wanted to explore her concerns in the most efficient and quickest way possible. She scored 4 (poor) on the emotional chart. The clinician was surprised at the high score having anticipated that her score would not indicate an unusual level of emotional dysfunction. The information was forwarded to her regular clinician.

Case 9: A man in his late 30s was seen by his clinician for back pain. It was a chronic problem, yet the patient would report only periodically to the practitioner when he "felt it was necessary." The injury resulted from a motor vehicle accident. The patient was frustrated because he "was not healing quickly enough." He was asked to complete the COOP charts. He scored his emotional health as poor (5); amount of pain as moderate (4); indicated that his social function was hampered quite a bit (4); felt the change in condition had become a little worse; and that his overall condition was fair (4). The clinician reported that the extent of the man's pain and dysfunction became more apparent with the use of the charts. The patient was able to use the charts as a "tool to stress his problems to us." There was a positive effect in the management plan of the patient. An X-ray was taken and he was being followed on a more regular basis until the problem could be minimized.

Case 10: A young man in his late 20s was seen by a COOP clinician for the first time. The patient had no known chronic problems. He complained of severe chest pains. Upon reporting to the office he was asked to complete the nine COOP charts. He reported that he was able to do very heavy (1) physical activities; had some difficulty (3) with role; social function was slightly hampered; experienced moderate pain (4); had quite a bit (2) of social resources; his quality of life had good and bad parts about equal (3); his overall condition was fair (4); and his emotional function had been extremely bothersome (5) to him. The practitioner indicated that the charts proved to possess "high" utility at this encounter and provided valuable information for both the doctor and the patient. Although the patient had experienced trouble at home, he was unaware that those problems might be the cause of his chest pains. The charts, as reported by the clinician, "quantified the importance of emotional stress to the patient."

Case 11: An elderly man was under treatment for severe rheumatoid arthritis. The doctor knew that he was "occasionally" depressed by his inability to accomplish tasks. His physical function score indicated that he was only able to do very light activities (5); experienced some difficulty (3) with his role; experienced moderate pain (4); and that his emotional condition had been moderately bothered (3) by his illness. Feedback from the clinician indicated that after probing the patient further he was surprised to learn "how much more depressed he got than I realized." The charts provided the practitioner "with a greater understanding" of the patient's emotional needs.

Case 12: A 64-year-old woman was under treatment for high blood pressure, rheumatism, and heart and breathing problems. She was asked to complete the charts. For the most part, her scores were in the low range, indicating good functional ability. Her physical score indicated that she was able to do moderate (3) activities; experienced slight (2) emotional dysfunction; some difficulty (3) with role; not at all (1) limited in her social function; recieved quite a bit (2) of social resources; and rated her overall health as good (3). However, she indicated that she was experiencing a moderate (4) amount of pain. The clinician, surprised by her high score, discovered the patient was experiencing abdominal pain for which she was subsequently treated.

Case 13: An established elderly female patient under treatment for hiatus hernia had fractured her ribs in a fall. The clinician had anticipated functional limitations but was "considerably surprised" by the scores she reported two weeks later. Her physical, emotional, and role scores were all between 4 and 5 (poor), yet, her social function score was 2 (slightly affected). He questioned the patient and discovered that prior to the fall she "had been putting on a brave face for the doctor" and was, in fact, "markedly depressed."

Case 14: An 87-year-old female patient was under her doctor's care for heart problems. Most of her scores indicated high functional ability. The patient indicated, however, that her physical activity level was 3 or moderate and that her overall health was 3 or good. The doctor, surprised by her self-assessment, questioned her further and discovered that the patient appeared to have a hearing dysfunction. Extensive testing was recommended.

Case 15: A young woman, 27 years of age, was under clinical care for diabetes and kidney problems. The clinician anticipated that her overall health was good. The physical, social function, overall condition, and quality of life charts, were administered and the patient indicated substantial dysfunction in all areas (3 or 4). The scores indicated greater dysfunction than the clinician had anticipated and thus provided a more accurate profile of the patient's functional health.

Case 16: An established, 81-year-old patient was being treated for multiple problems (diabetes, high blood pressure, arthritis, and heart). Despite the number of health problems, the clinician was surprised at the substantial level of dysfunction. She scored 5s (poor) on physical function, emotional function, overall condition, social resources, and quality of life. The practitioner questioned the patient and spent a portion of the encounter discussing available sources of support. Information from the charts gave the clinician an appreciably different understanding of the patient than he had previously had.

Case histories 17 through 21 were provided from clinical encounters in The Netherlands.

Case 17: A 73-year-old female complained of severe chest and arm pain. The pain was intensified during and after minimal strain. The clinician suspected coronary sclerosis but was unable to convince the patient to see a specialist. The woman was asked to complete the charts (Time 1). Her high scores (4 or 5) indicated severe dysfunction across all dimensions. Based on the chart scores, she agreed to see the specialist. The diagnosis was recorded as coronary sclerosis/angina pectoris for which she was treated. At a follow-up visit to the general practitioner (Time 2), her chart scores showed improvement in all areas. The following diagram illustrates the woman's functional health scores at the time of her initial encounter with the primary provider and after being seen and treated by the specialist. The improvement in self-reported scores shown below mirror those reported by her clinician.

	Physical function	Emotional function	Role function	Social resources
Time 1 {prior to specialist}	4–light	4–quite a bit	4–much difficulty	4–yes, a little
Time 2 {after specialist}	3–moderate	2–slightly	2–no difficulty	2–yes, quite a bit

Case 18: An established, 81-year-old female, under treatment for severe arthrosis of several joints, completed the charts at an initial encounter for a swollen ankle (Time 1). Her scores indicated severe dysfunction across all dimensions. Her ankle was treated and at the follow-up visit the charts were readministered (Time 2). Her scores showed a slight improvement. At

approximately two weeks later (Time 3), she again completed the charts and her scores showed marked improvement from Time 1 scores. A timetable of her scores is shown in the following table.

	Physical function	Emotional function	Role function	Social resources
Time 1 {Initial encounter}	5–very light	4–quite a bit	5–could not do	3–yes, some
Time 2 {Follow-up}	4–light	2–slightly	3–some difficulty	1–yes, as much
Time 3 {Two weeks later}	2–heavy	1–not at all	1–no difficulty	1–yes, as much

Case 19: An established, 79-year-old female was given the charts by her clinician. Her physical function appeared stable, but the patient reported substantial (a score of 5) emotional and social resources dysfunction. The doctor discovered that "she thought of herself as an absolute bore and therefore refused contact with family and friends." She was subsequently treated for depression.

Case 20: An established, 73-year-old, male patient was being treated for arthrosis and "different pain complaints." The practitioner reported that by using the charts, he discovered the patient was concerned about the problems he had with his son's wife and was "a bit depressed" about them. Alerted by information from the charts, the clinician surmised that the family problems, heretofore unrecognized, had a pronounced influence on the patient's health and the degree of pain he experienced.

Case 21: An established, elderly female patient under treatment for motor neuron disease and bulbar palsy was given the charts. Her physical, emotional, and social function score were all 5 (poor) and her role score was 4 (much difficulty). Her clinician, alerted by these high scores, was able to intervene and treat the patient for the depression that had gone unnoticed.

Common threads and findings

Case studies provided from 21 clinician–patient encounters demonstrate the clinical utility of the charts. The charts provided: better communication; discovery of new physical problems; discovery of new emotional problems; new information regarding degree of dysfunction; and modification of management plan (physical, mental, or social). The following table summarizes the specific areas of clinical utility for the COOP charts as documented across the 21 case histories.

Summary Table: Clinical utility of the COOP FHS charts area of utility.

Case Number	Patient type Old	New	Study site US	Neth	Better Comm	New physical problems	New mental problems	New under FX[a] severity	Modify Rx plan Phys	Men	Soc
1	×		×		×						×
2		×	×		×		×	×		×	
3	×		×			×		×	×		
4	×		×			×		×	×		
5	×		×				×			×	
6	×	×	×		×			×	×		
7		×	×					×	×		
8		×	×								
9	×		×		×		×	×	×		
10		×	×		×						
11	×		×		×		×	×			
12	×		×		×	×	×	×	×		
13	×		×		×				×	×	
14	×		×			×		×	×		
15	×		×					×			
16	×		×		×						
17	×			×				×	×		×
18	×			×		×					
19	×			×			×				
20	×			×	×		×				×
21	×			×	×		×	×			

[a] Functional.

9
Studies with the Dartmouth COOP Charts in General Practice: Comparison with the Nottingham Health Profile and the General Health Questionnaire

B. MEYBOOM-DE JONG and R.J.A. SMITH

Introduction

In order to assess functional status in primary care during consultations and housecalls a simple instrument is needed. In a study of morbidity and functional status of 5,164 elderly–65 years and older–the COOP charts developed by Nelson et al. were used. The reliability, construct validity, and clinical evidence supporting the COOP charts are reviewed in this chapter. Data were collected by means of four different self-administered questionnaires, all with four COOP charts. The elderly were randomly divided into four groups. Each group received one of four different questionnaire combinations at the beginning and at the end of the study year. Additionally 150 elderly received the same questionnaire 3 weeks after the second reponse. Overall, 66% of the elderly, answered and returned the same questionnaire twice; 132 elderly answered and returned the same questionnaire three times. The test–retest reliability of the charts, measured by Pearson's R, were good to excellent at a 3-week interval ($n = 132$) and good at a 1-year interval ($n = 3,393$), with the exception of the physical chart. Kappa coefficients were fair at 3 weeks and moderate at 1 year. The construct validity was evaluated by comparing the charts with the short-form RAND health measures for physical and psychological functions, with the 30-item general health questionnaire, a 10-item activities of daily living (ADL) index, and the 11-item loneliness scale. Convergent correlations were stronger than divergent correlations. Additionally the charts are mutually inter-related and show overlap.

Correlation of the charts with sociodemographic characteristics of the patients were low but in the expected direction. The clinical evidence, as shown

The content of this paper was originally prepared and presented for the closed meeting of the Classification Committee of WONCA, World Organization of National Colleges, Academies, and Academic Associations of General Practitioners/Family Physicians, in Calgary in October, 1988.

by function profiles of cough, shortness of breath, hypertension, osteoarthritis, cerebrovascular disorders, depression, acute bronchitis, and caring for ill partner, support the validity and clinical utility of the COOP charts.

The conclusion is that the COOP charts are a feasible way to assess functional status. If a score of 3 or higher is obtained, more precise instruments are recommended.

Status of the Elderly in The Netherlands

Though The Netherlands has the highest percentage of institutionalized elderly in Europe, 88% of Holland's aged are living independently in home situations, in their own homes, or in specially designed houses. Of the remaining 12%, 8% live in residential homes and 4% in nursing homes or other institutions (1).

The independent elderly and the elderly living in residential homes depend on their family physician for primary health care. Only old people who live in nursing homes have their own geriatrician. Health for the elderly is important, not as an end in itself, but as a means to live as self-directed and autonomously as possible. Because being able to function is apparently more important to the elderly than the absence of disease, it is functional status, rather than diagnosis, which determines whether an older person can live an independent, and fulfilling life (2).

It is the family physician's task to help elderly patients maintain their independence and autonomy, to prevent the decline of functional ability, and, when possible, to improve functional status. By functional status we mean the level of functioning in daily life, in which the consequences of ill health and diseases are reflected.

To study the relationship between specific complaints and diseases, on the one hand, and limitations of functional status, we have done a study of morbidity and functional status of the elderly.

Morbidity was recorded by means of the International Classification of Primary Care (ICPC), and functional status was assessed at every encounter by means of COOP function charts (3, 4). In this chapter we will address the following question: What is the reliability, construct validity, and clinical evidence supporting the COOP function charts?

Methods

Design of the Study

The study consisted of two parts:

1. In the prospective part of the study, over one year's time, 25 family physicians recorded all the encounters—both consultations and housecalls—with the elderly patients on their list. Morbidity was recorded

A. Physical Condition

During the past 4 weeks...

What was the most strenuous level of physical activity you could do for at least 2 minutes?

1. Heavy, e.g.
   Run
   Cycling against the wind
   Carry heavy bag of groceries

2. Moderate, e.g.
   Walk, fast pace
   Carry groceries
   Wash car

3. Light, e.g.
   Walk normal pace
   Cycling regular pace
   Vacuum cleaning

4. Very light, e.g.
   Walk slow pace
   Take bath or shower
   Wash dishes

5. Nearly nothing
   I am not able to do any light physical activity

B. Psychological Condition

During the past 4 weeks...

How much have you been bothered by psychological problems such as feeling unhappy, anxious, depressed, irritable?

1. Never

2. A little of the time

3. Some of the time

4. Most of the time

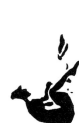

5. Always

C. Daily Tasks

During the past 4 weeks...

How much difficulty did you have doing your daily tasks because of your health problems?

1. No difficulty at all

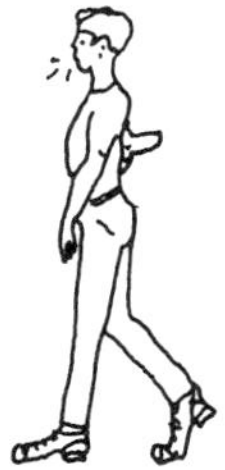

2. A little difficulty

3. Some difficulty

4. Much difficulty

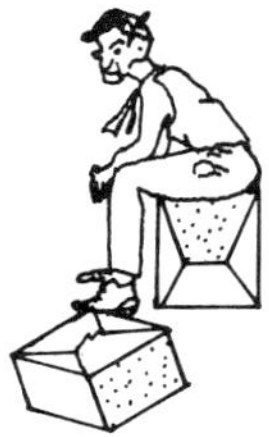

5. Could not do

D. Social condition

During the past 4 weeks...

How often have your health problems limited your normal social contacts with family, friends, neighbors, or clubs?

1. Never

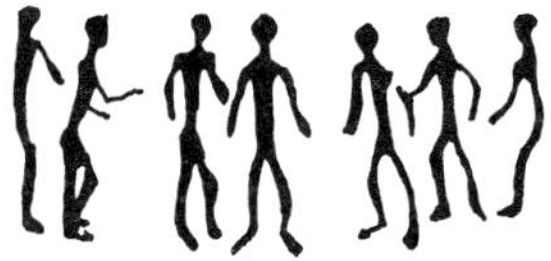

2. A little bit of the time

3. Some of the time

4. Most of the time

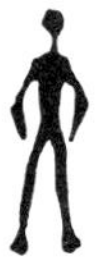

5. Always

FIGURE 9.1. COOP Function Charts

using ICPC, and functional status was assessed by means of the COOP function charts (Figure 9.1) (3–5).
2. By means of self-administered questionnaires, information concerning functional status was obtained from the elderly themselves, both at the beginning and at the end of the study.

Questionnaires

The following questionnaires were used in four different combinations:

LIST OF FUNCTIONAL ASSESSMENT

A combination of

1. Short-form RAND health status measures (6). Eleven yes/no questions on physical limitations, thirteen questions concerning psychological problems, for example, depression, anxiety, vitality (six possible responses). Five global questions about physical, psychological, and independent functioning (five possible responses) (5). COOP charts dealing with physical condition, psychological status, ADL, and social status (five possible responses). A low score indicates better function, a higher score more limitations. In the function profiles we combined the scores 4 and 5 to one score—serious limitations (4).
2. General health questionnaire (GHQ). Thirty questions dealing with mental health problems (four possible responses). Range of scores 0 to 15. Categories of scores: 0 to 4, no mental health problems; 5 to 8, possible mental health problems; $\geqslant 9$, definite mental health problems (7–9).
3. Nottingham health profile (NHP). Thirty-eight yes/no questions belonging to six subscales: energy, pain, emotional reactions, sleep, social isolation, and physical mobility (10, 11).
4. Activities of daily living. Ten questions of physical ADL (three possible responses). Range of scores, 10 to 30. Categories of scores, 10 to 16, ADL independent; 17 to 23, need help; $\geqslant 24$, dependent (12, 13).
5. Loneliness. Eleven questions dealing with feelings of being alone (three possible responses). Range of scores, 0 to 11. Categories of scores, 0 to 3, not lonely; 4 to 6 a little lonely; $\geqslant 7$, lonely (14).

Data Collection

At the beginning of the survey period, the elderly were randomly divided into four groups. Each group received one of the four different questionnaire combinations. Both partners of a married couple received the same questionnaire.

At the end of the year, the same questionnaire was sent to the groups who had responded previously.

Three weeks after that, the List of Functional Assessment, composed of the short-form RAND health status measures and the COOP charts, was sent again to the first 150 persons, who returned their questionnaires to assess the test—retest reliability of the charts over a relatively short period of time.

RELIABILITY

To study reliability, we used a test—retest strategy: The scores from the beginning and the end of the year were compared. Similarly the end-of-the-year scores were compared with scores from the last set of responses.

Two statistics, the Pearson's product—moment correlation and Cohen's Kappa, were used to measure levels of concurrence. The Kappa is a more rigorous test because it corrects for agreement due to chance. To provide consistency of interpretation, the following descriptive labels were given (15, 16):

Pearson's product—moment correlations: excellent, > .74; good, is .60 to .74; fair, .40 to .59 poor, < .40. Cohen's Kappa: nearly perfect .81 to 1.00; sufficient/good, .61 to .80; fair, .41 to .60; moderate, .21 to .40; poor, < .21.

CONSTRUCT VALIDITY

Validity deals with the question: How well does an instrument reflect that which it intends to measure?

Construct validity is the degree to which the "new" COOP function charts correlate with such other instruments of established validity as the GHQ, NHP, ADL, and loneliness scale.

For those questionnaires with more items per dimension, we computed a total score if the realiability coefficient of internal consistency (Cronbach's alpha) exceeded .80.

We assessed both convergent and divergent validity. In the presence of convergent validity, we expected to observe moderate to strong associations between corresponding dimensions. In the case of divergent validity, we expected weaker correlations between different dimensions.

We computed convergent and divergent validity by comparing the scores of the COOP charts with the other questions dealing with physical and psychological functioning from the short-form RAND health measures. Given the assumption that the GHQ, ADL, and loneliness questionnaires are valid and reliable, we computed the sensitivity and specificity of the COOP charts. For that purpose we made the following cross-tabulations:

COOP charts 1 to 5 × GHQ scores 0 to 4, 5 to 8, and $\geqslant 9$
COOP charts 1 to 5 × ADL scores 10 to 16, 17 to 23, and $\geqslant 24$
COOP charts 1 to 5 × Loneliness scores 0 to 3, 4 to 6, and 7 to 11

Clinical Evidence

Clinical evidence is the manner in which the empirical evidence from sociodemographic and clinical data supports the results of the measurements.

SOCIODEMOGRAPHIC VARIABLES

We computed the correlations of the COOP function charts with demographic characteristics:

Sex: male or female
Age: 65 to 100 years

Housing

1. own house
2. specially designed houses for the elderly
3. protected—living with children or in service flats
4. residential—living in residential homes

Socioeconomic status (SES)

1. unskilled labor (e.g., garbage collector)
2. skilled and trained labor (e.g., bus driver, carpenter)
3. "old" middle class (e.g., farmer, shopkeeper)
4. "new" middle class (e.g., teacher, white collar worker)
5. "higher status" class (e.g., manager, higher civil servant)
6. academic and upper class (e.g., physician, director)

DISEASES

One would expect that the diagnosis *hypertension* would be associated with less physical limitations than, for example, *other cerebrovascular disease* and that *depressive disorders* would be associated with more psychological limitations than physical problems such as acute bronchitis.

To illustrate our clinical evidence, we computed a function profile for several complaints (e.g., cough and shortness of breath) and for several episodes (e.g., hypertension, osteoarthritis, cerebrovascular disease, depressive disorders, acute bronchitis, and "caring for ill partner"). We reported the functional status scores for new contacts and follow-up contacts separately. For new contacts, each score refers to one new patient; for follow-up contacts, one patient can be responsible for more ratings. A patient in bad shape, who consults the doctor frequently, may rate his functional status more frequently and influence the total score in one direction. Also, co-morbidity, the number of episodes present in one patient, influences the functional status score.

Results

Population Characteristics and Responses

At the beginning of the study, questionnaires were sent to 5,164 elderly patients, of whom 4,039 (78%) responded. At the end of the year, 3,393 of the 4,039 elderly (84%) answered and returned the second questionnaire. Only small differences in demographic characteristics were found between respondents and the population at large: among the respondents there were slightly more women, more health-insured people, and fewer people living in a residential home. Overall 66% of the elderly returned both questionnaires, and 132 of 150 elderly (88%) returned three questionnaires.

RELIABILITY

The test–retest correlation between the ADL charts at three weeks was excellent and, of the remaining charts, the correlations dealing with physical condition, psychological status, and social contracts were good (Table 9.1). This suggests that the charts results are stable over relatively short periods of time. Correlations at one year were good except for physical condition, of which the correlation was fair. Lower correlations (one year versus three weeks) are expected, since changes in function may well occur over this longer time-span. Kappas were fair at three weeks and moderate at one year.

CONSTRUCT VALIDITY

In Table 9.2 the mutual correlations between COOP charts, global questions, and the other questionnaires are shown. The pattern of the first survey and that of the second survey are similar.

The physical chart correlated well with the ADL questionnaire and poorly with the loneliness scale and the emotional reactions and social isolation scale of the Nottingham health profile. Apparently the physical chart measures something that is seldom captured by the other instruments.

The psychological chart correlated well with the global questions on psychological function, the total score of the 13 psychological questions of the short-form RAND Health status measures, and the GHQ. This chart correlates poorly with the pain scale, the social isolation scale and the mobility scale of the Nottingham health profile.

It is evident that the ADL chart correlates well with all the other questionnaires except with the loneliness scale and the Nottingham health profile.

The social chart correlates well with the total score of the psychological questions of the short-form RAND health status measures and it correlates

TABLE 9.1. Test–retest reliability of COOP Charts at three weeks ($n = 132$) and at one year ($n = 3,393$).

COOP Charts	Pearsons correlation		Kappa	
	(3 wk)	(1 yr)	(3 wk)	(1 yr)
1. Physical conditions	.67	.36	.50	.33
2. Psychological status	.73	.70	.52	.38
3. Activities of daily living	.82	.72	.59	.36
4. Social contacts	.74	.69	.49	.31

TABLE 9.2. Correlations between the scores of questionnaires (1st time 1st row; 2nd time 2nd row).

1	2	3	4	5	6	7	8	9	10	11	12	13	14	15	16	17	18	19	20
COOP Charts																			
1. Physical condition	.32	.46	.38	.53	.50	.32	.31	.52	.59	.38	.60	.18	.32	.44	.23	.19	.21	.21	.44
	.33	.54	.43	.58	.56	.36	.36	.58	.69	.43	.67	.21	.36	.48	.28	.20	.25	.19	.56
2. Psychological status		.56	.54	.46	.46	.70	.66	.41	.39	.77	.38	.36	.60	.42	.22	.31	.37	.29	.24
		.55	.55	.45	.46	.71	.69	.41	.39	.79	.33	.37	.62	.41	.24	.40	.39	.28	.28
3. Daily activities			.64	.72	.70	.60	.59	.66	.64	.67	.65	.29	.61	.60	.42	.29	.33	.29	.51
			.65	.73	.73	.62	.62	.69	.66	.69	.66	.30	.62	.58	.45	.38	.35	.26	.58
4. Social contacts				.59	.57	.55	.55	.53	.52	.61	.55	.36	.58	.45	.28	.29	.30	.34	.38
				.60	.59	.56	.56	.57	.54	.63	.53	.33	.58	.50	.31	.37	.31	.31	.45
Global Questions																			
5. Physical functioning last month					.84	.55	.55	.76	.75	.59	.73	.28	.54	.61	.35	.24	.27	.26	.57
					.84	.54	.54	.77	.77	.60	.75	.27	.56	.60	.39	.33	.33	.26	.66
6. Physical functioning now						.55	.56	.73	.71	.59	.70	.26	.53	.60	.36	.25	.30	.28	.54
						.56	.57	.74	.72	.61	.70	.28	.54	.56	.40	.31	.32	.24	.61
7. Psychological functioning last month							.85	.48	.44	.79	.40	.35	.67	.45	.23	.37	.36	.34	.28
							.89	.52	.47	.81	.43	.34	.71	.47	.27	.51	.41	.34	.36
8. Psychological functioning now								.49	.44	.75	.42	.31	.64	.44	.23	.36	.36	.30	.28
								.52	.46	.78	.42	.34	.71	.48	.26	.51	.41	.34	.35
9. Independent functioning									.77	.54	.77	.23	.51	.58	.35	.22	.25	.26	.59
									.78	.57	.77	.23	.55	.57	.35	.31	.26	.27	.64

	1	2	3	4	5	6	7	8	9	10	11	12	13	14	15	16	17	18	19	20
Total Scores																				
10. Physical functioning (alpha = .91)											.52	.86	.25	.45	.64	.39	.29	.35	.33	.68
											.52	.86	.27	.47	.61	.39	.28	.34	.27	.74
11. Psychological functioning (alpha = .95)												.48	.40	.74	.54	.31	.42	.44	.38	.34
												.48	.42	.78	.55	.30	.53	.48	.35	.41
12. Activities of daily living (ADL) (alpha = .90)														.44	.62	.36	.19	.27	.28	.64
														.43	.59	.37	.27	.25	.25	.74
13. Loneliness (alpha = .86)														.39	.21	.17	.29	.26	.45	.15
														.36	.21	.12	.26	.25	.41	.17
14. General health questionniare (GHQ) (alpha = .96)																				
Nottingham Health Profile (NHP)																				
15. energy (alpha = .73)																				
16. pain (alpha = .81)																				
17. emotional reactions (alpha = .67)																				
18. sleep (alpha = .73)																				
19. social isolation (alpha = .77)																				
20. physical mobility (alpha = .55)																				

only moderately with the loneliness scale and the social isolation scale of the NHP.

It is clear that the four COOP charts are mutually intercorrelated. Correlation of the ADL chart with the social chart is good; with the psychological chart and the physical chart, fair. The physical chart correlates only poorly with the psychological chart. Like health, functional status is a construct, that is, artificially split up in different dimensions. Although ADL overlaps with physical, psychological, and social dimensions, it appears that "physical" and "psychological" are more specific categories.

The physical chart shows stronger correlations with other measurements of physical function than with measurements of psychological function, and the psychological chart shows stronger correlations with other measurements of psychological function than with measurements of physical function. Convergent validity is characterized by stronger correlations among similar constructs than different constructivity (i.e., divergent validity) (Table 9.3).

From our cross tabulations, it appears that the best sensitivity of the COOP charts is obtained at a cut-off point between level 2 and level 3 (Table 9.4).

It is evident (Table 9.5) that the physical chart distinguished between people with ADL limitations and with mental health problems, that the psychological chart indicated people with mental health problems, and that the ADL Chart, too, indicated elderly with problems in daily activities, but to a lesser extent than did the physical chart. No chart showed an acceptable concurrence with the loneliness scale. The dimension *loneliness* is not captured by the COOP charts, and especially not by the COOP chart social contacts.

TABLE 9.3. Convergent and divergent validity.

COOP charts[a]	First time[b]		Second time[b]	
	Physical condition	Psychological status	Physical condition	Psychological status
CC physical condition	1.00	.32d	1.00	.33d
GQ physical functioning last month	.53c	.46d	.58c	.45d
GQ physical functioning this moment	.50c	.46d	.56c	.46d
TS physical functioning	.59c	.39d	.60c	.39d
Mean	.54c	.41d	.61c	.41d
Standard deviation	.05	.07	.02	.06
CC psychological status	.32d	1.00	.33d	1.00
GQ psych. functioning last month	.32d	.70c	.36d	.71c
GQ psych. functioning this moment	.31d	.66c	.36d	.69c
TS psychological functioning	.38d	.77c	.43d	.79c
Mean	.26d	.71c	.37d	.73c
Standard deviation	.03	.06	.04	.05

[a]CC, COOP Charts; GQ, global question; TS, total score.
[b]c, convergent validity; d, divergent validity.

TABLE 9.4. Cross tabulation: Psychological COOP Chart × general health questionnaire.

Psychological COOP Chart	General health questionnaire			
	> 9	5–9	0–4	Total
5	18	3	7	28
4	72	11	10	93
	──────A──────	──B──		
3	143	99	252	494
	────C────	───D───		
2	18	29	388	435
1	6	14	585	606
Total	257	156	1,242	1,655

Cut-off point	Sensitivity	Specificity
A	35	98
B	25	99
C	91	73
D	25	78

TABLE 9.5. Sensitivity and specificity of the COOP Charts compared with the GHQ, ADL, and loneliness questionnaire.

COOP Chart	Questionnaire	Sensitivity	Specificity
Physical ×	GHQ	80	50
Physical ×	ADL	94	52
Physical ×	Loneliness	67	50
Psychological ×	GHQ	91	73
Psychological ×	ADL	69	84
Psychological ×	Loneliness	44	82
ADL ×	GHQ	73	87
ADL ×	ADL	76	84
ADL ×	Loneliness	66	96
Social ×	GHQ	71	85
Social ×	ADL	68	83
Social ×	Loneliness	51	82

Cut-off-point, COOP Charts between score level 2 and 3.

Clinical Evidence

The correlations between COOP charts and the demographic variables age, sex, housing, and SES are not strong but tend to go the expected direction (e.g., the physical chart shows a moderate correlation with age) (Table 9.6).

The function profiles that deal with the reasons for encounter show that functional limitations associated with shortness of breath are rated worse than those associated with cough (Figure 9.2). Shortness of breath is associated with serious physical limitations in 60% of the encounters, cough in only 30%. Shortness of breath is associated with serious limitations of ADL in 30% of the encounters, cough in only 12%. Shortness of breath and cough are associated with serious social interferences in 20% and 10% of encounters, respectively, and with serious psychological problems in 10% and 5% respectively. In

TABLE 9.6. Correlations between COOP Charts and sociodemographic variables (1st time, 1st row; 2nd time, 2nd row).

	Sex	Age	Housing	SES
COOP Charts				
1. Physical condition	.16	.40	.28	.07
	.20	.39	.25	.16
2. Psychological status	.18	.13	.14	.09
	.17	.10	.10	.10
3. Daily activities	.11	.23	.22	.08
	.12	.22	.19	.09
4. Social contacts	.10	.20	.19	.08
	.09	.17	.16	.11
Global Questions				
5. Physical functioning last month	.10	.33	.30	.11
	.12	.31	.25	.11
6. Physical functioning this moment	.08	.30	.26	.09
	.10	.26	.22	.10
7. Psychological functioning last month	.13	.13	.16	.08
	.14	.14	.16	.11
8. Psychological functioning this moment	.12	.15	.16	.11
	.12	.14	.14	.11
9. Independent functioning	.12	.35	.32	.10
	.10	.30	.27	.11
Total Scores				
10. Total score physical functions	.23	.44	.37	.13
	.22	.43	.33	.14
11. Total score psychological functions	.19	.15	.16	.12
	.18	.15	.16	.12
12. Total score ADL	.08	.49	.45	
	.06	.49	.43	
13. Total score loneliness	.06	.09	.11	
	.09	.12	.08	
14. Total score GHQ	.05	.13	.14	
	.06	.15	.12	
Nottingham Health Profile				
15. Energy	.44	.42	.60	.45
	.44	.40	.59	.43
16. Pain	.23	.22	.42	.28
	.21	.21	.40	.26
17. Emotional reactions	.19	.31	.29	.29
	.16	.29	.27	.28
18. Sleep	.21	.37	.33	.30
	.19	.35	.34	.29
19. Social isolation	.21	.29	.29	.34
	.19	.25	.27	.30
20. Physical mobility	.44	.24	.51	.38
	.44	.21	.47	.37

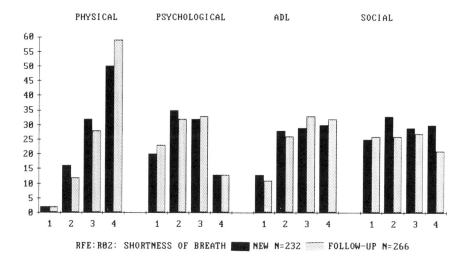

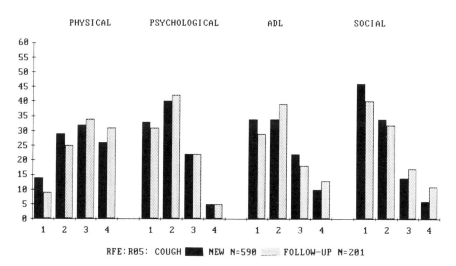

FIGURE 9.2. Function profile of reason for encounter:-shortness of breath (R02) and cough (R05) (1, unlimited; 2, slightly limited; 3, moderately limited; 4, seriously limited).

follow-up encounters especially, shortness of breath is associated with many physical limitations.

The function profiles of the episodes show a similar pattern (Figures 9.3 and 9.4): With the physical chart, serious limitations are assessed at most encounters; in about half of these cases "serious" limitations on the ADL chart,

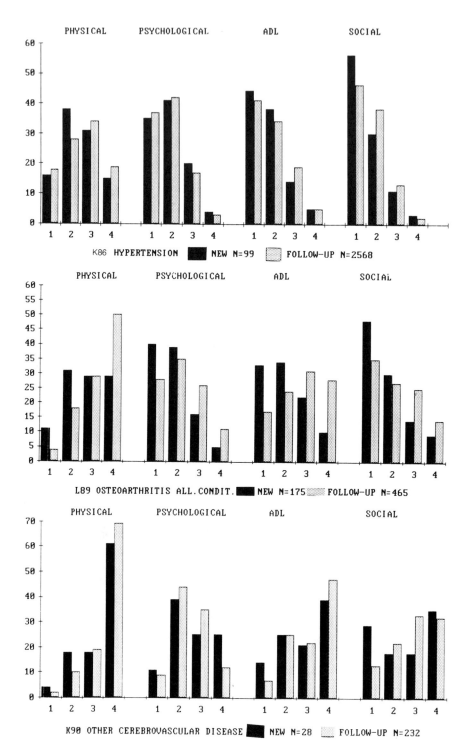

FIGURE 9.3. Function profile of hypertension, osteoarthrtitis, and cerebrovascular disease (1, unlimited; 2, slightly limited; 3, moderately limited; 4, serious limited).

146

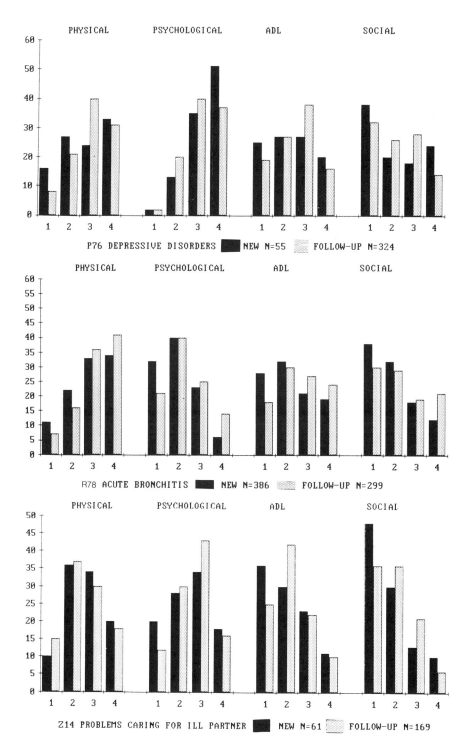

FIGURE 9.4. Function profile of depressive disorders, acute bronchitis, problems caring for ill partner (1, unlimited; 2, slightly limited; 3, moderately limited; 4, seriously limited).

and in half of these cases again there are "serious" limitations on the psychological and the social charts. Usually more serious limitations were assessed in follow-up contacts than in new contacts.

It is evident that hypertension was associated only slightly with serious limitations. Other cerebrovascular disease and osteoarthritis were associated with more serious physical limitations. In 70% of the follow-up contacts dealing with cerebrovascular diseases, serious physical limitations were assessed.

Depression, caring for an ill partner, and cerebrovascular diseases were more often associated with serious psychological problems. The physical chart showed more serious limitations than the ADL chart, perhaps because of the way the question was phrased. The physical chart was phrased positively: "What was the most strenuous level of physical activity you could do for at least two minutes?" Whereas the ADL chart was more phrased negatively: "How much difficulty did you have performing your daily activities because of health problems?"

Conclusions

COOP charts are feasible way to assess functional status. Their reliability is good. The physical chart and the psychological chart showed acceptable construct validity, as shown by fair to moderate correlations with other questionnaires of established validity.

The ADL chart overlaps both the physical chart and the psychological chart. This was expected because both physical handicaps and psychological problems interfere with daily activities. The social chart has both physical and psychological aspects. Interference with social contacts are a result of both psychological and physical limitations. One of the possible explanations is that no distinction was made between receiving a visitor and going out to visit someone. During the study, the participating family physicians remarked that patients rarely spoke up about difficulties in their social contacts. If the doctor knew, for example, that an elderly widow had relationship problems with her only daughter, it would take time and tact before she would speak about it. The question of the social chart on limitations in social contacts because of health problems is not specific enough. I would recommend splitting this question into three parts: having a confidant, receiving social support, and receiving a visitor. Is the social dimension indeed an external confounding variable, as Ware (17) stated in 1982?

In our view, the COOP function charts, as an entity, are a useful tool to screen and monitor functional limitations in elderly patients. The charts may improve health care in daily practice when used on certain types of patients at selected intervals.

We would like to thank E.G. Nelson for his critical comments.

References

1. Grundy E, Arie T: Institutionalization and the elderly. *Age Ageing.* 3:129–137, 1984.
2. Fillenbaum CG: *The Well-Being of the Elderly.* Geneva, World Health Organization, 1981.
3. Lamberts H, Wood M: *International Classification of Primary Care.* Oxford, Oxford University Press, 1987.
4. Nelson EC, Wasson J, Kirk J, et al.: Assessment of function in routine clinical practice: Description of the COOP Chart method and preliminary findings. *J Chron Dis.* 40 (suppl 1):55S–64S, 1987.
5. Nelson E, Conger B, Douglas R, et al.: Functional health status levels of primary care patients. *JAMA.* 24:3331–3338, 1983.
6. Brook R, Ware J, Davies-Avery A, et al.: Overview of adult health status measures fielded in RAND's health insurance study. *Med Care.* July 17 (suppl); 1979.
7. Goldberg D: Use of the general health questionnaire in clinical work. *Br Med J.* 293:1188–1189, 1986.
8. Goldberg D, Bridges K: Screening for psychiatric illness in general practice: The general practitioner versus the screening questionnaire. *J R Coll Gen Pract.* 37:15–18, 1987.
9. Wright F, Perini A: Hidden psychiatric illness: Use of the general health questionnaire in general practice. *J R Coll Gen Pract.* 37:164–167, 1987.
10. Hunt SM, McEwen J, McKenna SP.: Measuring health status: A new tool for clinicians and epidemiologists. *J R Coll Gen Pract.* 35:185–188, 1985.
11. Buxton M: The economics of heart transplant programmes: Measuring the benefits. In: Smith GT. *Measuring the Social Benefits of Medicine.* London: Office of Health Economics, 1983.
12. Davidoff D, Slater PE: Domestic care dependency in the aged: A total community survey in Israel. *J R Coll Gen Pract.* 32:403–409, 1982.
13. Staff of the Benjamin Rose Hospital: Multidisciplinary studies of illness in aged persons. II. A new classification of functional status in the activities of daily living. *J Chron Dis.* 9:55–62, 1959.
14. Jong-Gierveld J de, Kamphuis F: The development of a raschtype loneliness scale. *Appl Psychol Meas.* 9:289–299, 1985.
15. Fleiss, refered to in Powers SA: A pascal program that assesses the inter-reliability of nominal scales. *Educ Psychol Meas.* 45:613–618, 1985.
16. Landis RJ, Koch GG: The measurement of observers agreement for categorical data. *Biometrics.* 33:159–174, 1977.
17. Ware JE, Brook RH, Lohr KN: Choosing measures on health status for individuals in general populations. *Am J Public Health.* 71:620–625, 1981.

10
Assessing Function: Does It Really Make a Difference? A Preliminary Evaluation of the Acceptability and Utility of the COOP Function Charts

J.M. LANDGRAF, E.C. NELSON, R.D. HAYS, J.H. WASSON, and J.W. KIRK

Introduction

Despite the intuitive appeal of functionally oriented, health care management, the clinical utility of routine functional assessment remains questionable. The Dartmouth COOP project, a primary care research network, has developed a practical, reliable, valid Chart System for use in busy clinical practices. The goal of the current study was to assess its potential clinical utility and acceptability to patients and clinicians.

Physicians reported that for one out of every four patients seen (25% of 335 patients) the Charts led to new information and, for 40% of these patients, the Charts reportedly initiated a specific new management action. Clinicians provided 22 case histories illustrating the utility of the Charts. In 59% of these cases, the Charts directly enhanced communication and in almost 41% of the cases, they led the physicians to explore and diagnose new mental problems. In 55% of the cases, the clinician gained a greater understanding of the severity of patients' functional abilities, and in 80% of the cases, this understanding influenced management plans.

In addition to affecting the practitioner–patient relationship, preliminary results suggest that the Charts provide new and clinically important information. Overall, these findings demonstrate the need for more rigorous studies on the impact of functional assessment on health outcomes.

Problems

Two major stumbling blocks thwart the widespread adoption of routine functional assessment in clinical practice. First, although many physicians may embrace a functional approach to health care management (1), current measures require a substantial amount of administration time and/or scoring time and thus are not conducive for day-to-day use in the busy office setting. Second, although several studies support the use of standardized screening instruments (2,3), clinicians still need to be convinced that the use of the screening instrument improves the detection of important problems. Unfortunately, current investigations yield conflicting results and further augment physician skepticism. For example, measurable changes in patient health during treatment (4,5) and withdrawal of treatment (6) have been documented and simple measures of health status have been used to identify patients at risk for high utilization of medical care (7,8). Additionally, the use of standard instruments increases the detection of mental and physical disability when compared to "clinical judgement" (9,10). However, two recent studies in which the utility of health status measurement in clinical practice was examined yielded different results (11,12). One study used a screening instrument for mental health problems in ambulatory patients. Feedback of elderly patients' scores increased the likelihood of clinician attention to psychological morbidity (11). In the other study, when the results of a 34-item, functional status questionnaire were given to outpatient clinicians, no change in management was observed (12). Thus, the clinical utility of functional status measures remains questionable.

The Dartmouth COOP Project has been developing a functional assessment system for routine use in busy office practices. Recent studies demonstrate that the COOP Charts are reliable and valid (13–15). However, if the COOP System is to overcome the limitations of existing measures, it is critical that the Charts be efficient, easy to administer, clinically useful, and acceptable to both patients and clinicians. This chapter presents preliminary findings on the clinical utility and acceptability of the COOP Chart System.

Methods

Definition of the COOP Chart System

Our approach is called the "COOP Chart" System because it was developed by the Dartmouth COOP Project, a network of community practices that cooperate on research activities, and because the scales used to measure function are each displayed on a different chart. At the heart of the COOP System are four Charts that measure physical, social, and role functioning, plus emotional status. Additional Charts were developed for use based on clinical and research interests. There are a total of nine Charts in the current COOP system; three focus on specific dimensions of function, two on symptoms or feelings, and three on perceptions; one is a health covariate, (see Table 10.1).

The Charts are similar to the Snellen Charts that are used to screen vision quickly. Each Chart consists of a simple title, a straightforward question referring to the status of the patient over a one-month period, and five response choices. Each response is illustrated by a drawing that depicts a level of functioning or well-being along a five-point scale. In accordance with

TABLE 10.1. Overview of the COOP Chart functional and health status measures for adults.

Dimension	Function	Symptoms/Feelings	Perceptions	Health covariate
Chart name	Physical Daily work Social activities	Emotional Pain	Health change Overall health Quality of life	Social support

clinical convention, high scores represent unfavorable levels of health on each Chart. (High scores for social support indicate lower levels of support.) For example, the physical chart responses range from 1 to 5. A score of 5 represents the greatest degree of limitation. Appendix A reproduces the Charts.

The Charts are a single-item global measure and are not meant to replace existing instruments. Used correctly, the Charts allow practitioners to screen patients quickly and efficiently and to highlight those individuals who might benefit from a more comprehensive inquiry of functioning and health-related quality of life. The screening instrument should be used periodically to monitor the progression of chronic disease of a patient and to diagnose the onset of new disease.

Study Sites

This chapter focuses on preliminary investigations of the acceptability and potential clinical utility of the COOP Charts, as reported by 20 primary care physicians after seeing a total of 634 patients in Australia, Canada, England, Japan, rural New England (USA), and The Netherlands. The clinicians were supporting members of one of three medical research organizations: The Dartmouth COOP Project, The Netherlands Family Practice Network (NFPN), or the World Organization of National Colleges, Academies, and Academic Associations of General Practitioners/Family Physicians (WONCA).

Coop

Several small studies were conducted in the New England practices (a total of 11 physicians, 372 patients). Patients were randomly selected using a systematic method (i.e, every other patient). In one study, patients ($N = 312$) presented to their clinician after completing 4 to 9 Charts per patient. The clinician was aware of the patient's scores. In the other study, patients ($N = 60$) also presented to their clinician after completing 4 to 9 Charts; however, the clinician was unaware of the scores and was asked to readminister the Charts. All clinicians made use of the Charts in providing care in whatever way seemed appropriate, and at the conclusion of the patient encounter, they provided the investigative team with feedback about the utility of the Charts for that particular encounter (i.e., Did the Charts provide new or valuable information/initiate new management action/influence communication with the patient?). The researchers conducted debriefing interviews with these clinicians and the supporting staff who had used the Charts to provide more in-depth information on clinical utility. In addition, the patients completed post-visit questionnaires about the Charts' medical importance, clarity, and appeal.

NFPN

Dutch language versions of four of the COOP Charts (physical, emotional, role, and social support) were used for 253 patients in the rural area of Freisland, a northern county of The Netherlands. Patients were cared for by members of the NFPN. The family practice center consists of three clinicians, two men and one woman, who see approximately 2,500 patients (of whom 330 are elderly) per year. Chart scores, reason for encounter, diagnosis, and procedures were gathered on all patients during the course of one year. Clinicians were asked to complete a debriefing questionnaire about the administration of the Charts, patients' response to the Charts, and clinical incidents when the Charts provided valuable information or alerted the clinician to changes in patient functioning.

WONCA

Six clinicians used the Charts for a total of 59 patients in an effort to gain hands-on experience with a functional assessment instrument. (The COOP Charts were one of two instruments selected by the WONCA participants.) Patients were randomly selected using a systematic method (i.e., every other patient). Clinicians were asked to evaluate the ease of administering the COOP Charts and patient response to the Charts; they were also asked to indicate if the Charts provided new or valuable information, initiated new management action, or changed/influenced patient–doctor communication during the encounter. Open-ended comments were also solicited.

Evaluation Criteria

A comprehensive review of the reliability and validity of the Charts is presented elsewhere (13–16) and is beyond the scope of this chapter. In brief, the results indicated that the Charts are generally comparable in their ability to detect impact of disease (and demographic status) on patient functioning to longer instruments. Tests to determine reliability and validity were conducted at four sites: (i) the COOP, (ii) the Veterans Administration Outpatient Department (OPD) in White River Junction, Vermont, (iii) in the Free Clinic and University Outpatient Department at the Bowman Gray School of Medicine, and (iv) in three urban areas (Chicago, Boston, and Los Angeles). Table 10.2 summarizes the methods used to assess reliability and validity, as well as the overall results. If the COOP Chart System is going to be both used

TABLE 10.2. Summary of COOP Chart evaluative studies and results.

Place	Sample size	Evaluation goal	Results
COOP Primary Care Practices: New England	$N = 372$	Reliability	Range of k for all Charts = .37–.87 ($x = .66$)
		Validity	Range of r for all Charts = .54–.78 ($x = .65$)
		Acceptability	89% of the patients enjoyed use of the Charts 97% of the patients understood the Charts
		Clinical utility	In 25% of the patients, clinicians learned new information For 11% of the patients, the Charts sparked new management action 76% of the patients indicated that the Charts influenced communication with the clinician
VA Outpatient Clinic: Vermont	$N = 231$	Validity	Range of r for physical, emotional, role, overall health, social resources Charts = .51–.70 ($x = .64$)
		Test–retest reliability	Range of k for all Charts = .80–.97 ($x = .90$)
Bowman Gray Outpatient Clinic: North Carolina	$N = 51$	Test–retest reliability	Range of k for all Charts = .55–.90 ($x = .74$)
Medical Outcomes Study: Chicago, Boston, Los Angeles	$N = 2,374$	Validity	Range of r for Charts = .45–.70 ($x = .61$) Using RAND measures as a "gold standard" by which to compare the validity of the Charts, results indicate the charts are comparable to RAND measures in ability to detect impact of disease and demographic status on on patient functioning
Family Practices: The Netherlands	$N = 253$	Clinical utility	Preliminary findings indicate the Charts are sensitive to individual patient changes over time

and useful, then it is essential that the main users of the system (clinicians and patients), as consumers, judge it to be acceptable and clinically useful.

The indicators used to assess the acceptability of the Charts to practitioners and pateints were as follows:

Does the Chart System fit into office practice? Can the Charts be easily
  integrated into routine data collection.
How do clinicians and patients react to the Charts? Are the Charts easy to
  understand and answer?

The indicators used to assess the utility of the Charts to practitioners and
patients were as follows:

Do the Charts affect the communication, or topics discussed, between the
  patient and the clinician?
Do the Charts provide the clinician with new or useful information about the
  patient?
Do the Charts lead clinicians to initiate new management actions in the care of
  the patient?

Results

Patient-reported acceptability data and clinician-reported utility data presented in the following paragraphs are from patients and clinicians within the
Dartmouth COOP Project only. Case study data were provided by clinicians
within WONCA and NFPN and the COOP and are presented under a
separate heading—Case Studies of Utility.

Acceptability

The results showed that the Charts are viewed positively by patients and
practice staff. A total of 93% of the patients ($n = 225$) reported that they liked
the Chart illustrations and 86% of patients reported that the Charts were easy
to understand. According to nurses ($n = 5$), 89% of the patients enjoyed the
Charts and 99% of the patients understood the Charts. The Charts could be
integrated into practice flow without disrupting office procedures and four
Charts took approximately three to four minutes to complete (see Table 10.3).

TABLE 10.3. Acceptability of the COOP Function Charts.

Variable	Patients reported[a] (%)	Nurse reported[b]
Enjoyed use of the Charts	89%	89%
Liked the illustrations	93%	NA[c]
Found Charts easy to understand	86%	99%
Had time to complete four Charts	NA[c]	Three to four minutes

[a] $N = 225$.
[b] $N = 5$.
[c] NA, not available.

Clinical Utility: Patients' and Physicians' Ratings

Of the patients studied, 76% reported that the Charts influenced communication with their physician. Patients' rating of the effect of the Charts on communication was related to the sex of patients, such that 86% of males versus 69% of females reported that the Charts influenced their communication with the physician. Of the patients studied 89% reported that the information provided by the Charts was important for the doctor to know and 85% indicated that the Charts affected management actions. Most patients (74%) rated the Charts as useful: 10% excellent; 21%, very good; 43%, good; 23%, fair; and 3%, poor (see Table 10.4).

Physicians ($n = 5$) reported that for one out of every four patients (25%) seen the Charts led to new information, and for 40% of these patients, the Charts initiated a new, specific, management action. The impact of the Charts on physician–patient communication (as viewed by the physician) was rated Positive for 13% of the patients, No effect for 85% of the patients, and Negative for 2% of the patients.

Regression results on 147 patients seen by five different clinicians vis-à-vis the clinician's rating of utility of the Charts (i.e., scored high, medium, or low) showed that physicians' utility ratings are significantly related to (i) a physician's perception of the Charts' ability to provide new information; (ii) the individual physician who did the rating; (iii) poorer emotional function of the patients; (iv) poorer physical function of the patient; and (v) the physician's perception of the Chart's ability to influence clinician–patient communication positively.

Case Studies of Utility

The richest information regarding the clinical utility of the Charts came from debriefing interviews and questionnaires. In summary, the use of the Charts regularly provided important information for both new and established patients;

TABLE 10.4. Patient-rated utility of the COOP Function Charts.[a]

Variable	Frequency
Influenced communication with my clinician	86% (males) 69% (females)[b]
Provided important information for my clinician	89%
Affected management actions	85%
Usefulness of the Charts	74%

[a] $N = 372$.
[b] The difference between the groups was statistically significant.

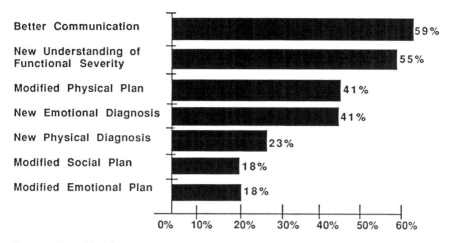

FIGURE 10.1. Clinician-reported utility of the COOP function and health status measures for adults.

frequently led to the discovery of previously unrecognized problems;
often revealed greater dysfunction in patients than had previously been
    recognized;
at times showed that the patient was functioning better than expected, given
    the disease status; and
improved communication between patients and clinicians.

Figure 10.1 summarizes the specific areas of clinical utility as documented
across 22 case histories. In 59% of the cases, practitioners indicated that the
Charts directly enhanced patient–clinician communication. Information
garnered from the Charts helped practitioners to explore and diagnose new
mental problems in 41% of the cases. In 55% of the cases, clinicians gained a
greater understanding of the severity of patients' functional abilities, and, in
most instances (80%), this understanding influenced the patients' management
plan. In particular, patients' physical treatment was modified in 41% of the
cases; in 18% of the cases, emotional treatment was modified; and in 18% of the
cases, social treatment was modified. As evidence of these findings, three case
studies are presented in the following paragraphs and three additional ones
are provided in Appendix B. Overall, these case studies begin to provide
evidence of the COOP Charts' sensitivity to changes in individual's health.

Case 1: A young man (37 years of age) with no chronic health problems was
seen by an emergency room physician for an injury to his finger. He saw his
personal physician a few weeks later for pain in his finger and arm and
reported having difficulty swallowing. The man was asked to complete the
nine Charts. His individual Chart scores are provided in the line graph below.
In general, his scores were high (4) and indicated poor levels of functioning.

Despite the fact that pain was the primary reason for this patient's encounter, he reported experiencing only "a very mild amount" (2). Upon further examination, the clinician learned that the injury, which had appeared quite trivial, was located in the patient's dominant hand. The patient had been unable to complete his usual tasks and activities. Arrangements were made for the man to receive Meals on Wheels. A month later the organic complaint had been relieved without the use of drugs. The patient reported feeling "significantly better," but he was still depressed. His "depression" complaint is being followed. The clinician indicated the most significant finding of the Charts was the wide-ranging extent of the patient's injury and the underlying emotional dysfunction.

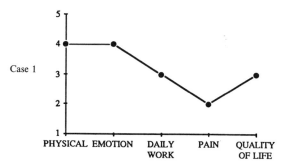

Case 2: A 62-year-old, divorced female was under treatment for palpitations, gastroenteritis, and diarrhea. She was well known to her clinician and had been a regular patient for many years. She was a quiet woman who "kept her chin up" and complained very little. Her clinician attributed these traits to her cultural background (Japanese). Her reported emotional score, however, revealed that she was "extremely bothered" (5) and this prompted the physician to take stronger measures to improve her emotional well-being.

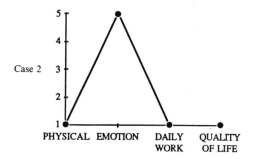

Case 3: An established elderly male patient (81 years of age) was under treatment for hypertension and arthritis and was well known by his clinician. During his clinical encounters the patient complained of fatigue and other nonspecific symptoms. He was married and devoted himself to the care of his

elderly wife who suffered from Alzheimer's disease. He received no family support and was unlikely to ask for help from others. The clinician characterized the patient as a very gregarious man who created symptoms so he could justify his regular visits to the office. The clinician reported difficulty accomplishing anything with the patient because he denied the root of his problems—he needed respite from the care of his wife. When evaluated with four COOP Charts—physical, role, emotional, and quality of life—the patient scored low on all measures, which suggested overall good health. The clinician knew that the patient's only outlet was visits to the office. He confronted the patient about the inconsistencies of his scores. Why was a man who reported good quality of life and emotional functioning frequenting the office as much as he did? Discussion with the patient revealed that Medicare had refused the man's request for respite because his wife was living in a stable home. The home conditions, however pleasant they were, taxed the patient. The clinician convinced the man to accept help and intervened with Medicare on his behalf.

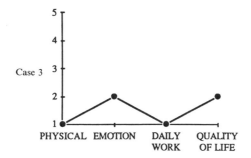

Discussion

These results on the acceptability and utility of the Charts are encouraging. First, the studies demonstrate that the Charts are easily integrated into the patient flow of busy clinicians' offices. This is a noteworthy accomplishment, since the majority of currently available health assessment measures were generated and refined in research settings. Second, patient response was favorable toward the Charts and patients indicated that the Charts provided valuable information to the practitioner. In the cited case histories, the Charts actually served as a communication vehicle for patient expression of health dysfunction. Third, the Charts frequently revealed substantially more dysfunction across all core dimensions than had been previously recognized by practitioners. The discovery of new physical problems occurred in only 5 of the 22 cases (23%).

This could be explained by several factors. Patients exhibit fewer untreated physical ailments or, due to the current orientation in medical education, clinicians are trained to treat organ systems and patients are socialized into the process of communicating physical problems. Patients are prompted to see a practitioner as the result of pain or discomfort; thus, during the natural course of most office visits, physical problems are more frequently revealed. Similarly, in general, physical treatment plans were modified in 41% of the cases versus 36% of mental or social treatment plans. However, it is important to be cautious about conclusions regarding modification of treatment. Much depends on the patient's reason for the encounter and the corresponding clinical diagnosis. Fourth, a qualitative analysis of the data reveals that the Charts opened two-way communication about topics that might otherwise have gone undiscussed. Overall case studies provide preliminary evidence that the Charts are sensitive to changes in the patient's health and provide clinically useful information. A large database plus a controlled trial are needed to document these claims fully. However, the value of single case studies, when every effort is taken to ensure accuracy and thoroughness, should not be underestimated.

In conclusion, the Charts provide a vehicle for both the patient and the practitioner to discuss areas of dysfunction that might have gone un-communicated despite the history-taking skills of the clinician. In addition to affecting the practitioner–patient relationship, the Charts can provide new, clinically important information and can assist practitioners to practice a style of medicine that maintains patients' abilities to function effectively in their natural environment. Overall, these findings demonstrate the need for more rigorous studies on the impact of routine functional assessment on health outcomes.

Acknowledgment. This work was supported by a grant from the Henry J. Kaiser Family Foundation of Menlo Park, CA (Grant Number 85-3180).

References

1. Cluff L: Chronic disease, function and quality care. *J Chron Dis.* 34:299–304, 1981.
2. Deyo RA, Inui TS: Toward clinical applications of health status measures: Sensitivity of scales to clinically important changes. *Health Services Res.* 19(3): 275–289, 1984.
3. Kane RA, Kane RL: *Assessing the Elderly*, New York, Lexington Books, 1981.
4. Sage WM, Hurst CR, Silverman JF, Bortz WM: Intensive care for the elderly: Outcome of elective and non-elective admissions. *J Am Geriat So.* 35:312–318, 1987.
5. Mackenzie CR, Charlson ME, DiGioia D, Kelley K: A patient-specific measure of change in maximal function. *Arch Int Med.* 146:1325–1329, 1986.
6. Walker FB, Novack DH, Kaiser DL, et al.: Anxiety and depression among medical and surgical patients nearing hospital discharge. *J Gen Int Med.* 2:99–101, 1987.
7. Wasson JH, Sauvigne AE, Balestia D, et al.: Capitation for medical care: The importance of health status in older patients. *Med Care.* 25(10):1002–1005, 1987.
8. Thomas JW, Lichtenstein R: Including health status in Medicare adjusted average per capita cost capitation formula. *Med Care.* 24(3):259–275, 1986.

9. Pinhold EM, Kroenke K, Hanley JF, et al.: Functional assessment of the elderly: A comparison of standard instruments with clinical judgement. *Arch Intern Med.* 147:484–488, 1987.

10. Davis TC, Nathan RG, Crouch MA, Bairnsfather LE: Screening depression in primary care: Back to the basics with a new tool. *Fam Med.* 19:200–202, 1987.

11. German PS, Shapiro S, Skinner EA, et al.: Detection and management of mental health problems of older patients by primary care providers. *JAMA.* 257(4): 489–493, 1987.

12. McDermott W: Absence of indicators of the influence of its physicians on a society's health. *Am J Med.* 70:833–843, 1981.

13. Nelson E, Landgraf JM, Hays RD, et al.: The COOP function charts: Single item health measures for use in clinical practice, in Stewart AL and Ware J (eds) *Measuring Functional Status and Well-Being: The Medical Outcomes Approach,* (in press).

14. Nelson EC, Berwick DM: The measurement of health status in clinical practice. *Med Care.* 27(3):577–590, 1989.

15. Nelson EC, Landgraf JM, Hays RD, et al.: Dartmouth COOP proposal to develop and demonstrate a system to assess functional health status in physicians' offices. *Henry J. Kaiser Family Foundation Final Report Grant # 85-3180,* October 1987.

16. Nelson EC, Wasson JH, Kirk JW: Assessment of function in routine clinical practice: Description of the COOP Chart method and preliminary findings. *J Chron Dis.* 40(S1):55S–63S, 1987.

Appendix A: The COOP Function Charts

PHYSICAL CONDITION

During the past 4 weeks . . .
  What was the most strenuous level
of physical activity you could do for at
least 2 minutes?

Very heavy, e.g. Run, fast pace Carry heavy bag of groceries upstairs	
Heavy, e.g. Jog, slow pace Climb stairs at moderate pace	
Moderate, e.g. Walk, fast pace Garden, easy digging Carry heavy bag of groceries	
Light, e.g. Walk, regular pace Golf or vacuum Carry light bag of groceries	
Very light, e.g. Walk, slow pace Drive car Wash dishes	

1

EMOTIONAL CONDITION

During the past 4 weeks . . .
  How much have you been bothered
by emotional problems such as feeling
unhappy, anxious, depressed, irritable?

| Not at all |
| Slightly |
| Moderately |
| Quite a bit |
| Extremely |

2

DAILY WORK

During the past 4 weeks . . .
  How much difficulty did you have doing
your daily work, both inside and outside the
house, because of your physical health or
emotional problems?

| No difficulty at all |
| A little bit of difficulty |
| Some difficulty |
| Much difficulty |
| Could not do |

3

SOCIAL ACTIVITIES

During the past 4 weeks . . . .
To what extent has your physical health or emotional problems interfered with your normal social activities with family, friends, neighbors or groups?

PAIN

During the past 4 weeks . . . .
How much bodily pain have you generally had?

CHANGE IN CONDITION

How would you rate your physical health and emotional condition now compared to 4 weeks ago?

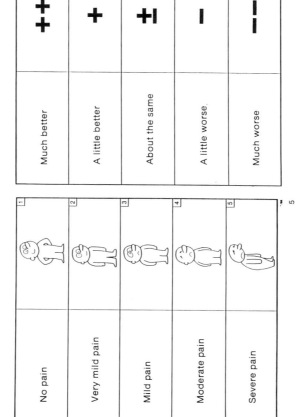

SOCIAL ACTIVITIES

Not at all	1
Slightly	2
Moderately	3
Quite a bit	4
Extremely	5

PAIN

No pain	1
Very mild pain	2
Mild pain	3
Moderate pain	4
Severe pain	5

CHANGE IN CONDITION

Much better	++	1
A little better	+	2
About the same	+‒	3
A little worse	‒	4
Much worse	‒	5

(continued)

Appendix A *(Continued)*

OVERALL CONDITION

During the past 4 weeks . . .
How would you rate your overall
physical health and emotional condition?

Excellent	1
Very good	2
Good	3
Fair	4
Poor	5

7

SOCIAL SUPPORT

During the past 4 weeks . . .
Was someone available to help you if you
needed and wanted help? For example if you

— felt very nervous, lonely, or blue
— got sick and had to stay in bed
— needed someone to talk to
— needed help with daily chores
— needed help just taking care of yourself

Yes, as much as I wanted	1
Yes, quite a bit	2
Yes, some	3
Yes, a little	4
No, not at all	5

8

QUALITY OF LIFE

How has the quality of your life been
during the past 4 weeks? i.e. How have
things been going for you?

Very well: could hardly be better	1
Pretty good	2
Good & bad parts about equal	3
Pretty bad	4
Very bad: could hardly be worse	5

9

COPYRIGHT © TRUSTEES OF DARTMOUTH COLLEGE/COOP PROJECT 1986
DEVELOPED WITH SUPPORT OF HENRY J. KAISER FAMILY FOUNDATION, MENLO PARK, CA, GRANT #85-3180

Reprinted with permission.

Appendix B: Case Studies—An Illustration of the Utility of the COOP Charts

The 3 case histories that follow (cases 1 through 3 are presented in the text) were selected from over 20 histories described by 11 clinicians during debriefing interviews and 9 clinicians using debriefing questionnaires.

Case 4: A clinician had assumed care for a 72-year-old patient with chronic obstructive pulmonary disease and angina. The patient had suffered a "small" stroke. The practitioner was "surprised" and "shocked" that the patient reported being severly limited in physical (5) and daily work (4) function. His high scores prompted the clinician to focus aggressively on the reason for the patient's low level of functioning. It was discovered Peripheral Vascular Disease (PVD) leg claudication had limited the patient's circulation and was responsible for his dysfunction.

Case 5: A young man in his late twenties was seen by a COOP clinician for the first time. The patient had no known chronic problems but he complained of severe chest pains. His Chart scores indicated that he was able to do very heavy (1) physical activities though he had some difficulty (3) with daily work and experienced moderate pain (4). His emotional function had been extremely bothersome (5) to him though he had quite a bit (2) of social support. The clinician indicated that the Charts possessed "high" utility at this encounter and provided valuable information for both the doctor and the patient. Although the patient had experienced trouble at home, he was unaware that those problems might be the cause of his chest pains. The Charts, as reported by the clinician, "quantified the importance of emotional stress to the patient".

Case 6: A 27-year-old woman, was under treatment for diabetes and kidney problems. The clinician viewed her overall health favorably, however, the patient indicated substantial dysfunction (3 or 4) in all areas (physical, social function, overall condition, and quality of life). The Charts provided the clinician with a more accurate profile of the patient's health.

11
Use of the Dartmouth COOP Charts in a Calgary Practice

R.C. WESTBURY

Introduction

Trials of psychometric instruments fall into the same category that the late Duchess of Windsor used for thinness and money; things that you can never have too much of.

At the time this trial was begun, the nine charts devised by the Dartmouth Medical School to measure functional status in family practice patients had already been tested in over 3,300 patient encounters. These trials had taken place in the United States and The Netherlands (1). They had shown that the COOP chart system was reliable, valid, and well accepted by both patients and physicians. Most of the early trials had taken place with selected patients. The developers emphasized that the charts were for quick screening, and seemed to suggest that their main use would be as a clinical tool to alert the physician to problematic functional status that might otherwise be missed. With regard to the psychometric properties of the charts, it was pointed out that they were "single-item global measures," to be considered individually, and that they were not to be used as a multiitem scale to obtain an index of functional status.

This trial arises out of the search by the Classification Committee of WONCA for a short instrument to measure functional status in family practice, one that is suitable for international use or that can be adapted for that purpose. In the past the committee has been involved in the development of classifications for international use in family practice: These have been primarily for use as research tools. It is envisaged that these classifications will interdigitate to form a system for the description of all the main elements of family medicine. So far there are classifications for (i) the presenting complaints of the patient, (ii) the reason for visit (the interpretation of the symptoms by the family physician before the patient is examined), (iii) the diagnosis or problems as the family physician sees them at the end of the encounter, and (iv) the ensuing process of investigation, follow-up, and treatment that is planned at the end of the encounter.

In order to complete the descriptions of what happens in family practice at this simple level, there is a need for a way to measure the outcome of all this activity by the patient and his family physician. The Classification Committee had decided that the best way to do this would be to have a measurement of the functional status of the patient from the subjective point of view, since this could be considered the "bottom line" for all medical activity. In essence this would be a measurement of "health status," but the hope was that by concentrating on how the patient functions, it would be possible to get a more reliable and comparable instrument, and to avoid the immense difficulties of defining health.

The committee looked at most of the systems of health or functional status measurements that have been devised so far and chose two instruments for further study: the University of Auckland Functional Assessment form and the charts from the COOP project at the Dartmouth Medical School. This study is of the latter instrument.

Method

The aim of this study was primarily to determine how the COOP charts would work if they were given to every patient seen. Family physicians are generalists in their practice, so there is a major need for research tools that can be used for the entire range of patients they see, from the perfectly well to the mortally ill. It was clear that it would be important to have the patients fill in the forms themselves if the goal of universality were to be achieved; if the doctor himself has to take the answers from each patient this would add 5 minutes to the average consultation time, an increase of 30 to 50% in the time spent with each patient. So the nine charts were reduced in size so that they could be presented to the patient on three sheets of paper. Instructions were printed at the top of the first sheet.

Although universality is to be desired, it was evident that there would be some patients who, for various reasons, would not be able to complete the form. The receptionist staff were instructed to prepare a form for every patient who came to the office, but not to give it to the following groups: (i) patients under the age of 15, (ii) patients who were very ill or in great pain, (iii) patients who obviously could not fill in a form for any other reason. If the patient refused to fill in the form, or failed to fill it in partially or completely, the receptionist was to record the major reason for this noncompliance. Receptionists were asked not to help the patients complete the forms; this rule was occasionally broken.

The COOP forms were changed in one way only. The original charts asked the patient to indicate his functioning in various ways over the period of one month. This was not appropriate when the patients were being asked to fill in the form at every list. Since the modal interval for follow-up appointments in my practice is about a week, the charts were changed to ask the patient how he had been feeling over the past week.

TABLE 11.1. Method for the physician's assessment of health rating.

Rules:	Consider patient's overall health at the beginning of the consultation
	Consider the most serious active problem
	Consider the presenting patient only

Classification:
1. Well. Presents for a non-illness reason
2. Illness or disorder of a trivial nature. No permanent sequelae are expected. Total resolution is to be expected within two weeks, with or without treatment. Little pain, discomfort, or disruption of life is involved.
3. Moderately ill. More severe than class 2, but lacks the possibility of death, severe discomfort, or disruption of life implied by class 4.
4. Very seriously ill. Death is a possible outcome at some stage, and/or extreme discomfort and/or major life disruption.
5. Mortally ill. Expected to die with one month.

For each encounter, the following information was also collected and entered onto the form: (i) the name of the patient, to allow me to get further information from the chart, (ii) the age of the patient, (iii) the sex of the patient, (iv) the social class of the patient. (This was recorded according to the well-known 5-point scale used in Great Britain) (2). (v) My own ad hoc health rating of the patient. (This is described in Table 11.1.) (vi) From April 14, the date of the encounter was recorded.

Results

Charts were prepared for 1,520 patients in the 25 weeks from March 14 to September 2, 1988. Of these, 330 forms were either not filled in at all or did not have answers for all nine questions. This left 1,190 fully completed forms for full analysis.

The distribution of the 1,520 patient encounters by age, sex, social class, and physician's health rating of the patients is shown in Figures 11.1 to 11.3. In

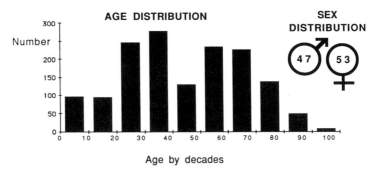

FIGURE 11.1. Age and sex distribution of the trial population.

Number of patients
in each class

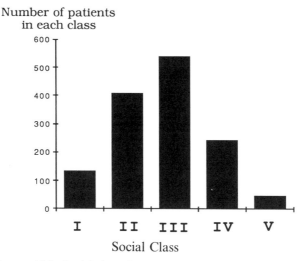

Social Class

FIGURE 11.2. Social class distribution of the trial population.

Percentage
in each category

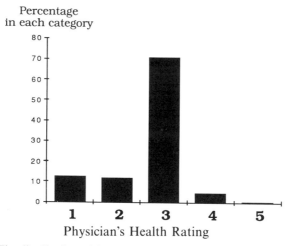

Physician's Health Rating

FIGURE 11.3. The distribution of the physician's health ratings in the trial population.

general, this distribution showed that the population tended to be skewed towards the older age groups, with 43.5% of the patient encounters being with people of age 50 or over; there is the common preponderance of females over males; it is an upper-middle-class practice, with 69% of the encounters taking place with middle-class patients. The distribution of degree of illness according to the view of the doctor shows the common pattern of a large preponderance of patients deemed to be ill enough to be concerned about, but not ill enough to be a cause of serious anxiety on the part of the doctor.

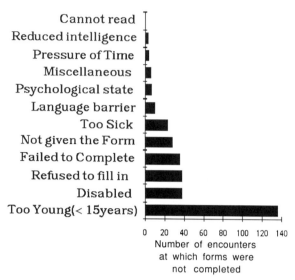

FIGURE 11.4. Distribution of reasons for not completing the forms.

Acceptibility

In all, 21.6% of the forms were either not filled in at all or had only some of the questions answered. Figure 11.4 shows the reasons for this rather high level of noncompliance. Young patients, under the age of 15, accounted for 8.9% of the full 1,520 encounters. The disabled were responsible for 2.5% of the forms not being completed, and the very ill another 1.5%. For 1.8% of the encounters, the staff did not remember to give the forms to the patient. Lesser reasons for noncompletion were language barrier (0.7% of visits), psychological state—this includes dementia (0.5%), the pressure of time (0.3%), and reduced intelligence (0.2%). Although it is estimated that 4% of Canadians are functionally illiterate, this was not identifed as a reason for noncompliance; it may well be that there were illiterate patients who managed to hide their disability behind one of the other labels. These figures do not take into account the many occasions when several of these reasons would seem to apply at once; only the most important reason was recorded.

In 38 cases (2.5%), the patient openly refused to complete the forms. Compared to all encounters, this was much more likely to occur with older patients (*t*-test; $p < .00001$) and with males (chi square; $p = .0001$). Failure to answer all the questions (2.4%) was more common in older patients, too (*t*-test; $p < .00001$), and was seen more often in females, but this association did not reach the level of statistical significance. One wonders if not answering all the questions may be the female pattern of resistance to the questioning.

Social class was not a factor in any of the major reasons for noncompliance.

It is interesting to examine the response patterns of these resistant patients at other visits. Although the numbers were too small to draw firm conclusions, it was noted that those who refused to complete the charts on one occasion were more likely to have actually completed them on a previous visit than they were to complete them on a visit subsequent to the visit at which they refused to comply. This suggests an element of "once bitten, twice shy." This is not unexpected with those who actually refused outright, but a similar pattern is seen in those whose reason for noncompliance is given as "Sick" and "Failed to complete all the questions"; it seems that these patients may really be refusing to comply but want to avoid a confrontation. The "Disabled" and the "Psychologically unfit" did not show this pattern. Both the "Sick" and the "Disabled" were more likely to score high on my health rating, confirming that I considered them to be more ill than the average patient (chi square; $p < .00001$ and $p = .06$, respectively), and were likely to be older (t-test; $p < .00001$).

Some patients filled in some but not all charts, and it was revealing to look at which charts were avoided. It was not a random process, as Figure 11.5 shows; there was a tendency for fewer questions to be answered the higher the number

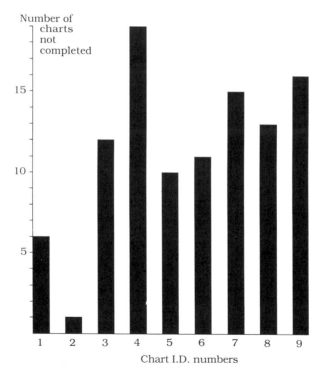

FIGURE 11.5. The number of times in the trial that each COOP Chart was not answered by a patient. (Note that the charts were administered in numerical order.)

of the chart as they worked their way through the form; in other words, these patients tended to be worn out by the effort. But two charts seemed, to be the exception to this rule: chart 4, social activities, was selectively avoided, and chart 2, emotional condition, was selectively chosen. Possibly the patients especially wanted to tell me about their emotions, but to talk of their social activities seems to have been either incomprehensible or distasteful.

Accuracy

Because of an anomaly in the arrangement of the questions, it was possible to check for one pattern of inaccurate answers that might be expected to be common. In all of the charts except chart 6, the "best" (i.e., least ill) response is answer number 1; chart 6 concerns change in perceived health, and answer 1 reads "Much better," whereas answer 3 is the more "normal" response, "About the same." Patients who want to get through the questionnaire as quickly as possible might be expected to read the first few questions, see that normal people would check answer 1, and then would check answer 1 for all subsequent questions. This only happened on five occasions; only three patients were responsible for this pattern of response, and all of them had been in for other visits at which they gave a less questionable pattern of answers. This suggests that these responses probably did truly reflect the state of health of the patients as they saw it, rather than indicating automatism. The only other instance of a straight set of identical numbers was one patient who answered "2" to every question: once again this patient gave a different answer at another visit.

There are no hard data on other possible systematic sources of error with the charts; one should consider the possibility that patients may not have understood some of the questions, or that they understood the question, but did not know how to answer, it. There is anecdotal evidence of the former difficulty in the comments offered by the patients.

Content Validity

Figure 11.6 is a diagrammatic representation of the relationship of the nine questions to the widely accepted "tripartite model" of family medicine. It would appear that there are some difficulties in matching the questions to this model. There is a tendency to cluster the questions around the biopsychological aspects of health and illness and to under-represent the contribution of social factors to well-being. One might characterize this as "being old-fashioned" or "thinking like a specialist," but it has to be admitted that, in reality, most family doctors still think like this most of the time. The three questions that do relate to the social dimension are all rather specific; charts 3 and 4 refer directly to the effect of bodily and mental health on just one aspect of social functioning... rather than the effect of social factors on the body and the mind for instance. Chart 8 focuses on one limited, though important aspect

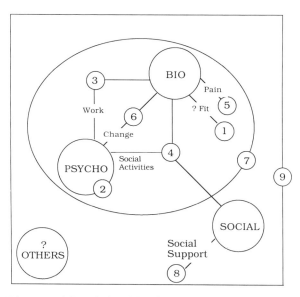

FIGURE 11.6. Diagram of the relationship of the content of the nine COOP charts to the tripartite model of family medicine.

of social function. The global questions are distributed rather unevenly: there is a global question about mental health, but not about general physical health, or about "social health." There is a question about the "universal" quality of life, but, as will be seen later, it is hard to link this very clearly with the other global questions.

Construct Validity

Figure 11.7 shows the percentage distribution of encounters for the sum of scores on charts 1 through 5 and 8 (summative score D) for patients at the five levels of health as judged by the doctor. The modal value tends to move towards the right of the graphs (i.e., the sicker end) as one moves down from the top graph of patients deemed to be without illness, to the bottom one of those considered to be mortally ill. This is evidence of construct validity, but one can see that there is considerable overlap of the graphs. The patients with the highest summative scores do not fall into the group of most ill patients as judged by the doctor, and the scores of the three mortally ill patients could be found on the top chart of patients who are thought to be perfectly well. This suggests that the summative scores lack discriminative power. The same pattern is seen if one plots the scores of any individual chart.

It should be emphasized that one would not expect a very good correlation between the doctor's health rating and the summative score—the correlation averages 0.25—for several reasons: (i) according to the developers of the

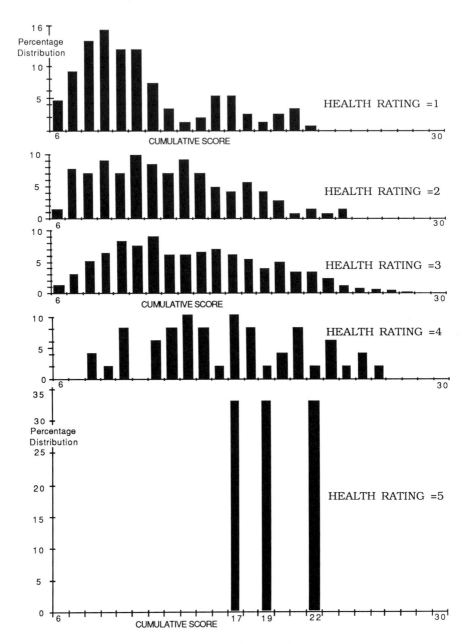

FIGURE 11.7. The percentage distribution of summative score D (6 charts) for each level of the physician's health rating.

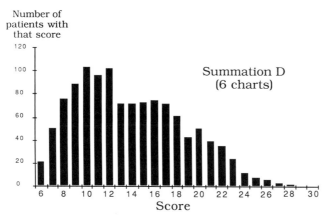

FIGURE 11.8. Overall distribution of summative score D.

COOP charts, one is taking a liberty in using summative scores. This will be discussed further below. (ii) It has already been shown (Figure 11.3) that the psychometric properties of my health rating are extremely poor. (iii) The reason we are searching for a subjective measurement of the patient's functioning is that we recognize that outsiders, even those with medical training, cannot say how the patient feels.

I have not had time to look at the progress of the scores on each chart for individual patients through time, as they get better or worse; this may demonstrate a better ability to discriminate... in this case between getting better or worse, rather than being ill or not ill.

The overall pattern of the distribution of the summative scores (Figure 11.8) fits with the expected pattern of a bell-shaped curve with positive skewing, reflecting the tendency of office patients to be only moderately ill.

Dispersion Patterns

The pattern of dispersion of the answers to the nine charts is illustrated in Figure 11.9. It can be seen that the patients tend to see themselves on average as being nearer to the well end of the scale as regards their quality of life (chart 9) than they do as regards physical health and emotional condition (chart 7), but, as Figure 11.10 shows, there is still a correlation between these two charts at the 0.64 level. This fits with what might be expected in the setting of family practice; "I feel rotten, but hell, I ain't complaining."

It is desirable to have a wide dispersion of answers to each chart, in order to maximize the sensitivity and discriminative power of the instrument. On this basis, charts 9, 6, and 7 should be reexamined.

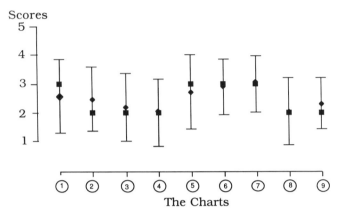

FIGURE 11.9. The pattern of dispersion of the answers to each of the nine charts. Guide to the symbols: The "feet"—one standard deviation from each side of the mean; the "diamond"—the mean; the "square"—the median.

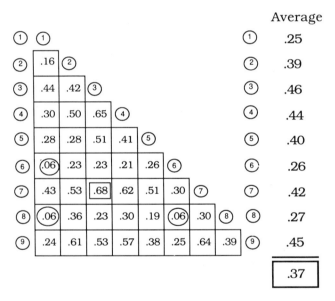

FIGURE 11.10. The intercorrelations between each of the nine COOP charts, the average intercorrelation for each chart, and the mean of those averages.

Reliability—Internal Consistency

Intercorrelations between the nine charts are shown in Figure 11.10. The level of these correlations is suprisingly high for single-item global measures; only three are very low at .06. These are limited to charts 1, 6, and 8. The next lowest correlation is 0.16, and the highest is 0.68; the overall average is 0.37, and it

FIGURE 11.11. The correlation between each of the nine COOP charts and summative scores A through D, and the mean correlation for each summative score. (The asterisks show which charts are in each summative score).

	A	B	C	D
1	*.80	*.66	*.61	*.57
2	*.71	*.67	*.63	*.65
3	.58	*.84	*.84	*.81
4	.52	*.79	*.77	*.76
5	.37	.50	*.71	*.68
6	.19	.24	.27	.26
7	.63	.76	.77	.76
8	.27	.31	.31	*.51
9	.54	.64	.64	.67
Mean	.51	.60	.64	.67

would seem that this could be raised considerably by either eliminating or modifying charts 1, 2, 6, and 8.

Several methods of summing the scores from individual charts were tried (Figure 11.11), from summing two charts—summative score A—to summing all of the charts except chart 6 (because it is arranged differently: see above) and the big global charts 7 and 9—summative score D. It can be seen that the more charts that are summed, the higher the mean correlation between the charts and the summative score. Obviously the correlations are higher for those charts that are part of the summative score, and this effect is more marked for the small sums; but two of the lowest correlations with summative score D are with charts that are part of the sum, charts 1 and 8. Again chart 6 shows a low correlation.

Patient Comments

The following were the commonest problems mentioned by the patients in speaking to me or in writing on the forms:

1. Difficulty in answering multiple embedded questions.
2. Difficulty in understanding the meaning of the maximum they "could do" in chart 1. I have the impression that chart 1 caused the greatest difficulty in understanding.

3. Problems of generalization: (i) over time, even though the period was reduced to a week for this study, and (ii) over health components as in charts 7 and 9.
4. Feeling constrained by the available answers; many patients either checked several answers or made the check mark in between answers.
5. There seemed to be considerable difficulty in grasping the reason for a functional status measurement. In the final analysis, although it is true that in 78.4% of the encounters the patient filled in the form as requested, I was struck by the fact that almost all of the spontaneous comments were negative, and a few were strongly hostile. I was surprised that the search for "A better way to ask 'How are you?'" was not understood and welcomed by more of the patients.

Discussion

This trial demonstrates that it is feasible to use the COOP charts on every patient at every office visit with this sort of population, provided that (i) the charts are self-administered and (ii) one is prepared to accept that as many as one in five encounters will not result in a usable result. It may be possible to reduce the failure rate by allowing the receptionist, the accompanying person, or the general physician to help the patient to complete the form, but each of these techniques would need to be independently validated and compared to the others. More energetic promotion of the form, and patient education about the value of functional status measurement, could also be expected to improve compliance.

It should be noted that this population was of higher social class than average and so was probably better educated and more sophisticated than many groups of patients. One wonders if the trial would have fared so well with a poorly educated rural population, to take one example.

This study confirms that the COOP charts show evidence of construct validity but strongly suggests that some charts are better than others. It would probably be possible to improve the instrument by either eliminating or modifying some of the questions. Charts 1, 4, 6, 7, 8, and 9 should be examined especially closely.

There is reason to question whether it is correct to consider that these charts represent single-item global measures, considering the rather high levels of correlation between the scores on some of them. Possibly there really is an underlying unifying theme to all these questions. It is tempting to wonder if this is not "health." If it were possible to add some questions, delete some others, and make changes in the wording of still others, so that the level of correlation was raised, it might be possible to gain the reassurance that comes with following classical psychometric theory for a homogeneous set of items.

The issues of multiple embedded questions and generalization need to be addressed. A case could be made for having the time frame of the questions less even than a week; possibly the last 24 hours might be more appropriate.

The wording of the questions in English needs to be re-examined critically. When the COOP forms are translated into different languages, problems will recur for each new language. Thought will need to be given also to the cultural premise on which the questions are based, as distinct from the words used.

The issue of sensitivity was only touched on here: it is a critical consideration for functional status measurement in family medicine. Since most of our patients are not very ill, the extent of the change to be expected is relatively small, and therefore more difficult to capture. Fortunately the high volume of patients and the continuity with which they are seen over time in our field are exactly the conditions needed to explore this neglected aspect of the technology of functional status measurement.

The meager evidence here suggests that the COOP instruments is low in systematic response bias, but this needs to be studied further. As the form is moved to international use, specific studies of the understanding and the validity of self-assessment for each chart will be needed.

Psychometric theory favors longer instruments containing more items: the difficulty is that the conditions of general practice make it very impractical to use forms that take more than about 5 minutes to complete. My receptionist estimated that most patients filled in the COOP forms within 5 minutes: it may be possible to add a few more questions. If this were to be done, then it would seem to be useful to include global questions to tap the fields of physical health in general and social health in general. Possibly there should be another question in the area of social functioning. Since the big global questions (charts 7 and 9) correlate rather highly with the summative scores, it would seem to be reasonable to eliminate them.

Chart 6 does not live up to the expectations suggested by common sense; it should be eliminated.

Both the patient comments and psychometric considerations of the importance of discriminative power and sensitivity in general practice suggest that it would be beneficial to increase the number of possible responses to each question. There is little practical advantage in having more than 11 possible responses for each question (3).

Conclusions

The COOP charts have many of the properties that the Classification Committee of WONCA are seeking, but much modification, clarification and testing will be needed even to meet the requirements of family practice in North America. To expand this work to satisfy family practice researchers in other cultural milieux will be an even greater task... one that is exceeded only by the need for such an instrument, and by our determination to meet that need.

References

1. Nelson EC, Landgraf JM, Hays RD, et al.: Dartmouth COOP proposal to develop and demonstrate a system to assess functional status in physicians' offices. Hanover, New Hampshire: Dartmouth Medical School, 1987 (Mimeo.).
2. Registrar General, England and Wales: *Classification of Occupations, 1960.* London, HMSO, 1960.
3. Nunnally JC: *Psychometric Theory,* 2nd ed. New York: McGraw-Hill pp. 595–596, 1978.

12
A Trial of the Dartmouth COOP Charts in Japan

H. SHIGEMOTO

Introduction

The affiliate hospital of Kawasaki Medical School in Japan first established the Department of Family Practice eight years ago. Six years ago they opened a walk-in clinic, without facilities for admission, in Kurashiki City, 6 kilometers from the affiliate hospital. The number of patients visiting for the first time exceeds 10,000 and 70 to 100 patients consult two physicians daily. A total of eight physicians bear the workload. The distribution of all patients by age and sex is given in Figure 12.1. The range of medical care covers almost all primary care areas, including internal medicine, ambulatory surgery, orthopedics, dermatology, pediatrics, total health care, and advice on life-style

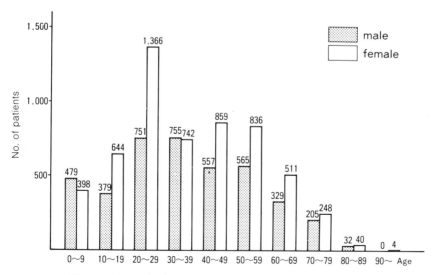

FIGURE 12.1. Distribution of age and sex (9,700 patients).

such as diet and physical exercise. Patients requiring admission to the hospital are treated by the clinic staff and other specialists.

A field test of the Dartmouth COOP charts was performed on 144 patients aged 18 and over with chronic diseases who were visiting for either the second or a subsequent time.

Methods

Patients independently completed nine charts in which they rated physical condition, emotional condition, daily work, social activities, pain, change in condition, overall condition, social support, and quality of life. The charts were completed prior to consultation with the physician and only a small number of aged people required help with the charts. Correlations between scores on the Dartmouth COOP charts and number of health problems, number of process items, and number of drugs prescribed were assessed.

Results

The distribution of the study group of patients by age and sex is given in Figure 12.2. In accord with the total patient population (Figure 12.1), the number of females exceeded that of males. Table 12.1 details the health problems found in the study group, in rank order of frequency. A total of 384

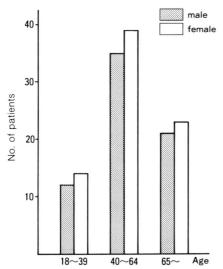

FIGURE 12.2. Distribution of age and sex.

TABLE 12.1. Health problem and its frequency.

	Number of cases	Percent (per 144 cases)
Hypertension	53	36.8
Diabetes mellitus	30	20.8
Iron deficiency anemia	24	16.7
Obesity	20	13.9
Hemorrhoids	17	11.8
Low back pain	16	11.1
Gastroduodenal ulcer	15	10.4
Chronic hepatitis	13	9.0
Gout	8	5.6
Cholelithiasis	8	5.6
Arthritis deformans	8	5.6
Osteoporosis	8	5.6
Heart disease	7	4.9
Total	384	(2.7 problems per one patient)

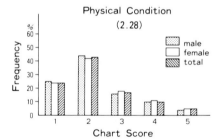

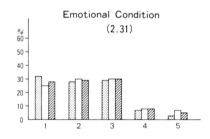

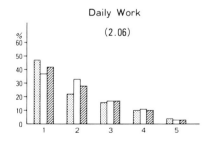

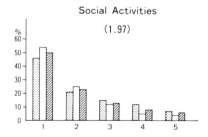

FIGURE 12.3. Frequency of chart score (1).

problems were recorded, for an average of 2.7 problems per patient. As expected for primary care adult patients, hypertension, diabetes mellitus, iron deficiency anemia, and obesity were most frequent.

The distribution and mean scores of the nine Dartmouth COOP charts is detailed in Figures 12.3 and 12.4. Lowest mean scores (low scores indicate less impairment) were attained for social activity and social support (1.97 and 1.73, respectively), while assessment of overall condition and quality of life (3.02 and 2.57, respectively) received the poorest evaluations.

Chart scores of patients, where N represents number of cases, with one or two health problems ($N = 71$) were compared with those of three or more

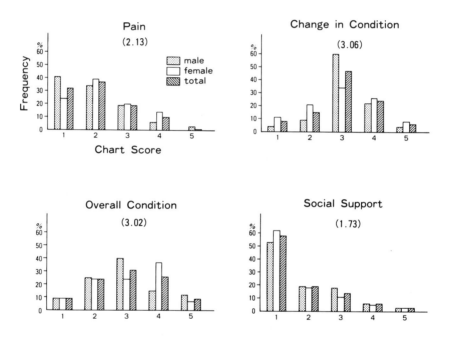

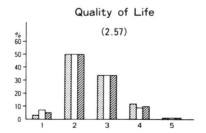

FIGURE 12.4. Frequency of chart score (2).

($N = 73$). Patients with fewer health problems rated physical condition, daily work status, social support, and quality of life better and described a more favorable change in condition then patients with three health problems or more. Differences in other chart scores were negligible. Thus it appears that an increased number of health problems is inversely related to functional status assessments (Table 12.2).

The IC-Process-PC (1) was used to record the process of medical care. Almost half of the patients received a clinical laboratory work-up, although some patients received two or more (Table 12.3). Because of the large number of chronic diseases in our patient sample, counseling and health education was also a frequent medical intervention. The second clinic visit often occurred soon after the first and the item health education (previously recorded) may therefore be underrepresented. Chest X-ray, upper gastrointestinal series, and abdominal echography were the most frequent tests included in the diagnostic imaging category.

Functional status also appeared to correlate with the number of process items given to patients (Table 12.4). With the exception of emotional

TABLE 12.2. Correlations between number of health problems and chart score.

COOP chart \ Health problems	1 ~ 2 ($N* = 71$)	3 ~ ($N* = 73$)
1. Physical condition	2.20	2.36
2. Emotional condition	2.35	2.28
3. Daily work	1.92	2.22
4. Social activities	1.93	1.90
5. Pain	2.11	2.11
6. Change in condition	3.17	2.79
7. Overall condition	3.06	2.99
8. Social support	1.61	1.82
9. Quality of life	2.42	2.62

*N = number of cases.

TABLE 12.3. Process in patient care and its frequency.

Process	Number of cases	Percent
Clinical laboratory	174	49.3
Diagnostic imaging	47	13.3
Other diagnostic procedures	25	7.1
Therapeutic procedure	9	2.5
Counseling and health education	94	26.6
Referral to a specialist	4	1.1
Total	353	100

condition, poorer functional status was noted in patients who received four tests or more as compared with those who received less than four tests. The difference between scores on emotional function were negligible between the two groups.

With the exception of those charts that measure social function, there was a linear relationship between function and the number of medications prescribed for patients (Table 12.5). Those patients taking four or more drugs reported better physical and emotional conditions, daily work, less pain, improvement in condition, and better overall condition and quality of life than those taking less than four drugs; yet our clinic physicians attempt to reduce polypharmacy and almost none of the patients in the study group was receiving six or more drugs. Improved function could be the result of effective drug therapy or may relate to a longer period of attendance at the clinic.

TABLE 12.4. Correlations between number of process and chart score.

COOP chart	Process	$0 \sim 3$ ($N = 83$)	$4 \sim$ ($N = 61$)
1. Physical condition		2.12	2.48
2. Emotional condition		2.23	2.18
3. Daily work		1.96	2.23
4. Social activities		1.81	2.13
5. Pain		2.08	2.18
6. Change in condition		2.92	3.16
7. Overall condition		2.88	3.28
8. Social support		1.59	1.80
9. Quality of life		2.45	2.62

TABLE 12.5. Correlations between number of drugs and chart score.

COOP chart	Drugs	$0 \sim 1$ ($N^* = 55$)	$2 \sim 3$ ($N^* = 47$)	$4 \sim$ ($N^* = 42$)
1. Physical condition		2.95	2.26	2.05
2. Emotional condition		3.20	2.43	2.02
3. Daily work		2.15	2.11	1.88
4. Social activities		2.13	1.72	2.02
5. Pain		2.24	2.11	1.95
6. Change in condition		3.40	2.87	1.62
7. Overall condition		3.24	2.91	2.86
8. Social support		1.51	1.74	1.83
9. Quality of life		2.96	2.43	2.55

$*N$ = number of cases.

Summary

1. Patients come self-administer the Dartmouth COOP charts in a brief period of time.
2. The cost of chart administration is minimal.
3. The picture-aided questions were easily understood by our patients.
4. The charts appeared to facilitate doctor–patient communication.
5. The nine charts produce a comprehensive picture of functional status.
6. Physicians in ambulatory clinics frequently neglect the assessment of functional status. These charts may be better administered on the second visit rather than the first because the required medical tasks at the second visit are frequently less than those at the first.
7. The information on change in functional status is useful to the patient as well as the physician.
8. Physicians are able to ascertain differences between their own assessment of functional status and that of the patients. Our physicians noted two problems with the Dartmouth COOP chart: (i) The chart assessing overall condition appears to be superfluous because its content is contained in the other charts and (ii) repeat administration produced different scores. It is uncertain whether this reflects a change in condition or inadequate reliability of the method.

Reference

1. Classification Committee of WONCA: *International Classification of Process in Primary Care* (IC-Process PC). Oxford, Oxford University Press, 1986.

Part IV Other Functional Assessment Instruments

13
Results of Studies of the Auckland Health Status Survey

S.R. WEST

My introduction to the WONCA Classification Committee was at the Singapore World Conference in 1983 when Bert Bentsen persuaded me to talk about my health status measures. In Tietlingen and again in London, we discussed the idea of a classification of function, not qualified by "health," and the consensus was that it should ideally be short enough to fit within the time constraints of family practice consultations. An instrument such as we had used for community needs surveys in Auckland was considered to be too long, too wide ranging, and too concerned with future health.

My own view is that health status measures will take many years to indicate *all* facets of health and that comprehensive health index scores will be possible only within small homogeneous groups (if such exist). However, I believe we can recognize an extensive mosaic of health states and influences that can be measured individually, validly, and reliably. The difficult part is to relate them quantitatively to each other and to know how they can be appropriately weighted when grouped.

In order to understand the relationships between measures, I suggest we look at the Functional Health Mosaic (Table 13.1) we find useful in Auckland. On the chart provided you will see, on the left, a list of basic abilities and needs. As you look to the right you see various stages and examples of personal development and sophistication of function right through to the peak performances of our best scholars, athletes, artists, models of healthy living, philosophers, and saints. (All the peak qualities will rarely be seen in one person, though Yehudi Menuhin, for example, has several.) We have filed lists of functions that can be objectively measured and we can also identify the people and the processes that aid movement in each direction.

This theoretical model has complemented, first, the expressed concerns of informed lay people and of key professionals (family doctors, public health, well-baby and district nurses, ministers of religion, social workers, and others) and, second, the results of community health-need studies conducted by household surveys, morbidity diaries, and enquiries addressed to special groups such as adolescents and the elderly. The questionnaire that evolved covers the areas of personal characteristics, enjoyment of life, vulnerabilities to

TABLE 13.1. Functional health mosaic (West).

	1 Basic biological needs	2 Basic living functions	3 Creative living functions	4 Peak performance
Inherent abilities				
Sensory ability	Vision Hearing Touch Smell Taste Postural balance Sensory coordination	Basic ability to learn Concentration Comprehension Recall	Intellectual creativity Thought Information–collection –organisation –analysis –integration –synthesis Problem-solving Planning Articulate Aesthetic/artistic appreciation	Intellect and judgment Artistic performance
Motor ability	Bones/joints Muscles Voluntary nerve system Involuntary nerve system Nerve-muscle balance Other body effects	Basic mobility and dexterity Walk Eat Dress Speak Write Get help Other daily living activities	Quality motor skills Posture Balance Fine control Dexterity Endurance	Physical performance
Visceral organ competence	Visceral organ function	Balanced organ functions	Artistic expression Energy level (physical)	Peace of mind
Environment-related needs				
General physical needs	(Supply and quality) Food Water Shelter Warmth Safety Rest	Good living environment Diet Hygiene Housing Clean environment Some life choices Health care Resources/access Employment	Positive physical health Physical state Health risks & prevention Health practices Health knowledge Health supports Quality services	Communication performance Social expression
General emotional spiritual needs	Gratification Loving care	Good emotional/spiritual environment Love & loved Self-respect Good personal relations Spiritually aware Sexually at ease Basic freedoms Sense of achievement	Positive enjoyment, social and spiritual expression Emotional/enjoyment state Personality Family interaction Philosophically/spiritually active Socially/culturally aware Social support system Social/spiritual health	Emotional/spiritual expression

health enhancement and breakdown, illness, disability, and health service utilization. This is therefore a list of health influences derived from grass-roots concerns and observations and related to a theoretical structure.

In order for us to evaluate our work objectively, we need to learn how to quantify the functions of patients. Some years ago our government set up a workshop on prescribing on the assumption that we prescribe too much. The fact is that we do not know if we over prescribe because we do not measure the effects of medication on our patients in holistic terms. Some of you will remember that, in London, I showed you a method of selecting tests to quantify the effects of treatments on patients dying of cancer.

I also demonstrated a pyramid model that is useful to demonstrate to medical students and others the diversity of health status items. This can be represented in a flat target form; see Table 13.2. The four pyramid sides, or target quadrants, respresent abilities, enjoyment, vulnerabilities, and a combination of supports and disease process. Each of the 32 segments contains up to five selected contributing items, which usually can be assessed objectively or subjectively. There is nothing wrong with subjective opinions founded on good observation and mature judgment when objective measures are not available. The model lets us to see at a glance the greatest deficits in comprehensive health at any assessment time so that we can direct attention to the highest priorities.

Because it is evitable that it is going to come up, may I say now that I am totally committed to the comprehensive view of patients' health, including enjoyment of life, the social environment, and the shaping of today's behaviors for the sake of future health. The family doctor must be the observer of the whole patient and his/her environment, and in most countries, the doctor is the gatekeeper to health and social services.

The Study Itself

The instruments used in the study were the pyramid chart of health assessment to supply descriptive headings for doctors and a health status questionnaire for patients (see Appendix). The purposes were to see

if doctors can assess patients comprehensively using their present knowledge;
if patients' opinions on their health and health-related matters differ from their doctor's opinions;
if, by seeing patient responses to the questionnaire, doctors learn more about patients and modify their own assessments; and
if items on the questionnaire and the chart change during the course of an illness so that progress can be measured quantitatively.

TABLE 13.2. Personal pyramid of health assessment.

Name: _____

							Exc.	Normal (For age and environment)		Not good		Poor		Very poor	Comments* prior[1]
							1	2	3	4	5	6	7	8	

Ability-disability

Personal self-care	Bathing	1–8	Toileting	1–8	Eating	1–8	Dressing	1–8			Opinion on mean
Home activities	Food preparation	1–8	Laundry	1–8	Housework	1–8	?Gardening	1–8	?Shopping	1–8	Opinion on mean
Task organization	Logic	1–8	Problem solving	1–8	Lateral thought	1–8	Integration of ideas	1–8	Fantasy	1–8	Opinion on mean
Mobility-dexterity	Movement in bed	1–8	Transfer (bed/ chair/other)	1–8	Walk (?with aids)	1–8	Fine movement	1–8	Hand grip	1–8	Opinion on mean
Communication	Vision (except simple lenses)	1–8	Hearing	1–8	Speech	1–8	Writing	1–8	Comprehension	1–8	Opinion on mean
Seeing place in world	Time-, Place-, Orientation	1–8	Personal Relationships	1–8	Active interests	1–8	Events enjoyed	1–8	Outings enjoyed	1–8	Opinion on mean
Perception of own health	Very good	1	Good	2	Fair	2	Poor	4	Very poor	6	Select one 8
Pain limiting	Severity		Duration		Frequency		Coping ability				General opinion

Emotional-enjoyment

Personality coping traits	Persistence	1–8	Everyday problems coping	1–8	Looks forward	1–8	Relax and enjoy	1–8	Moods	1–8	Opinion on mean
Enjoying activities	At Home	1–8	With family/friends	1–8	At work/school	1–8	In social contacts	1–8	In recreations	1–8	Opinion on mean
Life events last year/present	Death in family	4–8	Severe illness in family	4–8	Personal breakup	4–8	Change in job, home	4–8	Now: Most days Good/Bad	4–8	Opinion on mean
Cultural/social adaptation	Language		Cultural identity		Health attitudes		Land identity		Socioeconomic environment		General opinion
Intellectual function	Intelligence	1–8	Concentration		Attention span		Confusion		Psychiatric illness		General opinion
Basic psychological needs	Loving	1–8	Being loved	1–8	Sense of achievement	1–8	Self-respect	1–8			Opinion on mean
Spiritual/philosophical outlook	Religious faith	1–8	Secure philosophy		Self-sufficient		Yoga/TM/other				General opinion
Contentment/happiness	Usual aura										General opinion

Group	Attribute	Copes with severe stress (1)	Copes with moderate stress (2)	Not coping with modest stress (4)	Usually "stressed" (6)	Always "stressed" (8)	Select one
Vulnerability	Drive/stress	Copes with severe stress	Copes with moderate stress	Not coping with modest stress	Usually "stressed"	Always "stressed"	Select one
	Alertness/activity	Enthusiastic/Exuberant (1)	Bright/Active (1)	Subdued/less active (2)	Withdrawn/ bed/chair (4)	Unconscious/bed immobile (6)	Select one (8)
	Health history	Family predisposition (1-8)	Congenital problem (1-8)	Personal history; No problems (2-8)	Personal history; Transitory problems (2)	Personal Significant for future (2-3)	General opinion (4-8)
	Preventive care/education	Use of preventive practices (1-8)	Use of preventive services (1-8)	Education Formal	Education Health knowledge (1-8)	Education re health services (1-8)	Opinion on mean (1-8)
	Basic health needs	Water/Food/Shelter (1-8)	Hygiene/Sleep (1-8)	Sexual expression	Basic freedoms (1-8)	Self environment (1-8)	General opinion (1-8)
	Cultural & social influences	Diet (1-8)	Living conditions (1-8)	Violence exposure (1-8)	Cultural dissension (1-8)		General opinion
	Work influences	Occupational risks (1-8)	Job mortality risk (1-8)	Personal relations at work (1-8)	Responsibility at work (1-8)	Unemployment (8)	General opinion (8)
	Socio-economic influences	Income (1-8)	Educational status (1-8)	Occupational status (1-8)	Family type (1-8)	Ethnic: Known risks (1-8)	Opinion on mean (1-8)
Support	Family support (supplied/expected)	Relationship(s) (1-8)	Number of contacts (1-8)	Frequency (1-8)	Quality of support (1-8)		Opinion on mean
	Friend support "	Relationship(s) (1-8)	Number of contacts (1-8)	Frequency (1-8)	Quality (1-8)		Opinion on mean
	Professionals available "	Professionals available	Nature of support	Number of contacts	Frequency of contacts	Quality	General opinion
	Cohesion in network	Communication	Coordination				General opinion
	Receptive to help?	From aids or medicines (1-8)	From people (1-8)				Opinion on mean
	Economic security	Full range of choices (1)	Moderate range (3)	Limited (4)	Poverty (8)	Feeling of security (3)	Select one
Disease process	Noxious influences	Disease virulence	Trauma degree	Severity of attack	Risk to life	Risk to future health	General opinion
	Resistance to insult	Physiological resistance	Immunological resistance	Psychological resistance	Will to recover		General opinion

¹PTO indicates comments can be written on the opposite side of the page. Their presence is indicated by an asterisk (*).

The Responses

Nine of our members responded, from seven different countries. Fifty-seven patient questionnaires and original doctors' assessments were received, the number from each doctor varying from three to nine. Twenty-nine second doctors' assessments were completed after the doctor had read the completed patient questionnaire. One patient in Japan was assessed during a hospital admission and after discharge in order to monitor changes in health status items.

The instruments were supplied in English, which meant time-consuming interpretation of the patient questionnaire in two countries and the selection of English-speaking patients in a third. Our Canadian host prepared a commentary page to explain the New Zealand peculiarities I had inadvertently left in, and he elicited a helpful patient response.

General Comments

One doctor respondent accepted the overall concept but found the mechanism unmanageable, and this reduced his response. Some doctors had difficulty interpreting patient questionnaire responses in order to change them onto scores to fit the Pyramid Chart. (It was not intended that doctors do it.)

Not all respondents happily accepted the inclusion of questions about employment and work conditions, other life-style risks, religious or philosophical beliefs, or sexual expression. Some admitted to little knowledge of their patients' social supports. One commented that the questions had too much or too little specificity and provided little or no new knowledge— though the discrepancy analysis tended to refute this comment. There was an adverse comment on the inclusion of wellness as well as illness and on a lack of relevance to "daily tasks to find out why patients seek advice, what they suffer from, and how I can help them." There were constructive comments on some individual questions but little consensus in these.

All in all, one respondent was enthusiastically supportive, one solved a difficult long-term problem by using the questionnaire, three rejected the idea or the instruments as useful, and four made no general comments but complied with the process.

Analysis of Results

Fifty-seven paired responses, comprising the doctor's original chart assessment and the patient's completed questionnaire were received. Eleven percent of the items on the charts could not be compared because questions had not been completed, by either the patient or the doctor.

Discrepancies between the initial doctor assessment and the patient reports on each item were recorded if the scores differed by at least two grades or if a difference of at least one grade straddled the line between grades three and four, which determined whether a problem existed. In considering the first six headings for daily living activities, the patient was asked only to indicate if a problem existed, so any doctor's score within the problem grades (four to eight) was accept as congruent.

The last heading, referring to resistance to (disease) insult, was not usually assessable by the patient and no comparison could be made.

Let me say now that the questions to the patient were in a well-tried format, that differed from the cryptic headings the doctor was responding to. This could have led to some, though relatively few discrepancies.

(I would be happy to explain reconciliations between the patient questionnaire and the chart if you wish it.)

Question 1: Can doctors assess their patients comprehensively, using their present knowledge?

Doctors could assess their patients quantitatively and some scored almost all the 142 items on the chart separately. That two doctors completed only three patient assessments was due to excessive work load in one case and rejection of the process in the other. Some doctors commented that they were sometimes guessing in giving scores but their scores seemed reasonably accurate.

Question 2: Do patients' opinions on their health and health-related matters differ from their doctors' opinions?

Using the discrepancy criteria above, the patients' gradings differed from the doctors' in 29% of all questions. Among the assessments of daily living activities, personal self-care (bathing, dressing, etc.) had the least discrepancies (14%), but estimates of mobility–dexterity and communication differed between the doctor and the patient in 35% and 53%, respectively. Forty-nine percent of the doctors opinions about the patients' own perceptions of their health were inaccurate, as were 35% about the pain/discomfort suffered.

There was considerable variation between doctors. Two or three made very similar assessments of their patients in the first four questions about daily living activities and it would be interesting to know if that was related to the level of home visiting.

In the emotional–enjoyment section, discrepancies in scores for heading subjects varied between 20% and 49%, with an average of 35%. Some doctors seemed much better informed than others about the state of mind of their patients.

In the vulnerability section, discrepancies varied from 22 to 56% and averaged 37%. In considering health influences, the presence of significant disease in the past often, surprisingly, did not produce scoring appropriate to the description "significant for the future." Work influences were not as well estimated as expected, but this may have been due to the age of many subjects.

A 42% discrepancy occurred between socioeconomic influence scoring by the doctor and scoring by the patient.

Opinions about patients' supports showed better congruence, being closest for the professionals viewing themselves (15%) and widest for support from friends (35%). Opinions about family support differed in 24% of the replies. Economic security, like socioeconomic influences reports, was less well known by doctors.

The disease process enquiry was not scored consistently considering the health history, and congruence in opinion was 55%. I believe this subject is important and will require more attention and study in the future.

In total we see 29% discrepancy between doctor and patient opinions. Some assessments are higher for patients than doctors and some are higher for doctors than patients. For instance, the direction of discrepancies in patients' perception of their own health are almost equally divided. In general I would suggest that abilities and enjoyment are best judged by patients, vulnerabilities by doctors, and supports by both. The disease process is definitely a doctor thing and requires clarification. I believe a combination of opinions is helpful in all areas of enquiry for educational, if not evaluative, purposes.

Question 3: After seeing their patients' responses to the questionnaire do doctors change their scores?

Twenty-nine second round scores were provided, although some doctors did not provide any. The time interval between first and second doctor assessments was not recorded and there was some indication that changes in actual health status had occurred between assessments, and not that patient questionnaire results were influencing the doctor.

The revision of opinions was varied in direction and degree, with only a small tendency to move towards the patients' opinions! However, the one question one would expect patients to have an absolute say about was in their perception of their own health. Of the 29 reports of a second assessment, 18 (62%) scores exactly as the patient did, 6(21%) differed by one grade, 3(10%) by two grades, and 2(7%) by three grades. Do we find it so difficult to accept our patients' perceptions? Only one of our respondents scored *every* patient as the patient reported on this question.

Question 4: Can serial assessments be used to monitor the progress of patients, in functional terms, during an acute illness?

Dr. Shigemoto took the trouble to assess a woman patient 50 years of age who had hypertension and had suffered a stroke 9 months earlier. She had been admitted to hospital with headache and dizziness. We have no assessment before admission, but we do have a follow-up assessment after discharge. In the target version of the pyramid (Figure 13.1) in which the centrall bulls-eye is "exceptionally good" and the perimeter the "worst function," you see the assessment during admission in the dotted line and the postadmission

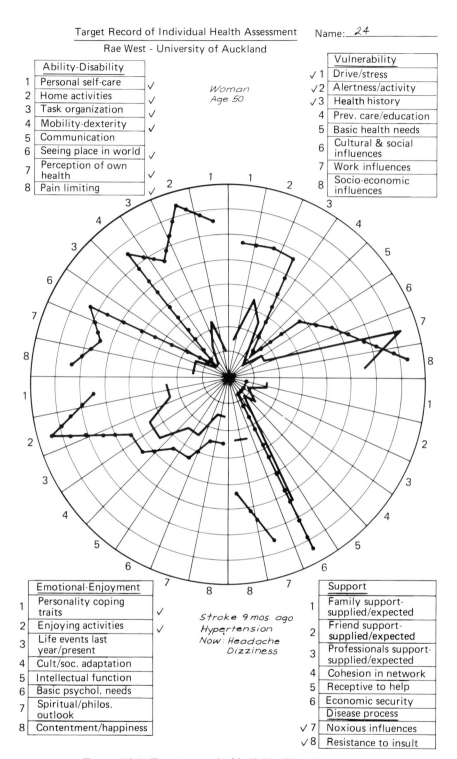

Target Record of Individual Health Assessment   Name: 24

Rae West - University of Auckland

	Ability-Disability	
1	Personal self-care	✓
2	Home activities	✓
3	Task organization	✓
4	Mobility-dexterity	✓
5	Communication	
6	Seeing place in world	✓
7	Perception of own health	✓
8	Pain limiting	✓

Woman
Age 50

	Vulnerability	
✓ 1	Drive/stress	
✓ 2	Alertness/activity	
✓ 3	Health history	
4	Prev. care/education	
5	Basic health needs	
6	Cultural & social influences	
7	Work influences	
8	Socio-economic influences	

	Emotional-Enjoyment	
1	Personality coping traits	✓
2	Enjoying activities	✓
3	Life events last year/present	
4	Cult/soc. adaptation	
5	Intellectual function	
6	Basic psychol. needs	
7	Spiritual/philos. outlook	
8	Contentment/happiness	

Stroke 9 mos. ago
Hypertension
Now: Headache
Dizziness

	Support	
1	Family support- supplied/expected	
2	Friend support- supplied/expected	
3	Professionals support- supplied/expected	
4	Cohesion in network	
5	Receptive to help	
6	Economic security	
	Disease process	
✓ 7	Noxious influences	
✓ 8	Resistance to insult	

FIGURE 13.1. Target record of individual health assessment.

199

(recovery) assessment in the plain line. Wide differences between the two assessments within segments demonstrate those states or functions that vary during an acute illness. These include all daily living activities except communication, and also perception of health and discomfort. In the enjoyment quadrant, personality traits and enjoyment-of-activities scores showed wide discrepancies. In vulnerability, initiative, alertness/activity and health history showed wide variation. Finally, as expected, disease process assessments varied as the patient recovered.

Summary

This project must be considered a descriptive feasibility study.

The project was insufficiently prepared because of unavoidable demands on my time and I accept responsibility for this. Response was limited in the number of respondents and, to some degree, by the numbers of cases per respondent. Analysis was limited by omissions in the completion of records. I understand the reasons for these limitations and I am grateful for the time given to responses.

Conclusions

The results of the survey suggest paying particular attention to the following principles:

If we are to be truly professional and wish to develop a respected role in the communities we serve we must put our traditional disease-care role alongside and not ahead of the comprehensive and preventive care we speak of but do little about. We must know more about the problems and potential influences on the health of our clients. Comprehensive data collection is made feasible by using patient time for questionnaires and record clerk time to screen information for the doctor's attention.

The results of the study suggest we pay attention to the following headings:

1. *Individual questions and tests* need further validation when used for different purposes. (One of our New Zealand Medical Research Council committees has adopted health status as a special interest. An experienced social scientist will complete a review of the literature and the feasibility of practical use in our country and she will report on it early in 1990.)
2. *The functional health mosaic* can be used to relate tests within the pattern of overall human development.
3. *Opinions are needed from both patients and doctors*, and whether from one or both for specific items of information should be studied further.
4. *Subjective assessments* by mature observers can be used until the objective aspects are worked out.

5. *A clear definition for potential use* is needed for specific items and groups of items as they relate to patterns of health needs in patients.
6. *A comprehensive measure* needs to include the quality of life, whole-patient functions, and preventive care.
7. *The outcome of care* should be measurable in functional terms and applied to all aspects of health care.
8. *Priorities for home and institutional care* should be determined on the basis of comprehensive functional assessment.

Finally, I must state clearly that the Auckland health status instruments are designed as comprehensive, practical, primary health care tools to indicate the precise needs for care and the precise responses we, as family doctors, have the power to make. If that is what the Classification Committee wants as the framework of a classification, I believe these measures, can contribute to this endeavor.

Appendix

<u>HEALTH SURVEY - CONFIDENTIAL LINK FILE</u>

Please complete the following :-

Family Name   _____

Address   _____

Phone Number

In the space below please write the first name, age and sex
of all the people who usually live in your house.
(If the family name of anyone in your house is different
from that written above please write their full name)

FIRST NAME (Put own name first)	AGE IN YEARS	SEX

FAMTYPE

□

FAMOCC

□

FAMED

□

HEALTH STATUS SURVEY

ADULTS QUESTIONNAIRE (P)

(for persons 16 years and over)

INSTRUCTIONS FOR COMPLETING THIS QUESTIONNAIRE

Please put a tick in the box or boxes which answer the question best

for you. Some questions require a brief written answer.

CONFIDENTIALITY: We recognise that much of the information in the

completed questionnaire is private. Please be assured that your answers

will be kept completely confidential. No names or addresses or information

that can be identified with any individual will appear in any report.

We require your name only so that we may contact you if you have missed

out any questions

PERSONAL
SERIAL

1.   Name _____|_____

            (first)   (family)

2.   Sex   Male ☐   Female ☐   ☐ SEX

3.   Age in years   ☐   ☐ ☐ AGE

4.   How long have you lived in your present district?

      (In contact with the same local people, shops and other

      services) _____   ☐ TIME

5.   Which ethnic group do you feel your family (or you if alone)

      belongs to most?

                                                                            ☐ ETHNIC

            Specify_____

6.   Which of these <u>best</u> describes your main state of employment?   EMPTIME

    (Tick one box)

    Full-time paid ☐   Looking after home and family full-time ☐

    Part-time paid ☐   Looking for work (including unemployment ☐
                              benefit)

    Voluntary work ☐
    (No pay and   On Benefit or Superannuation and not
    excluding home   working (other than unemployment benefit) ☐
    duties)
                     School or other student ☐

7.   What is your <u>job or occupation</u>?   PERSOCC

    (Please describe your occupation fully e.g. <u>dental</u> nurse, <u>auto</u>
    electrician. If retired or unemployed please say so and give   PERFAMOCC
    your previous occupation e.g. retired construction foreman)

_____

8. (a) How much education have you had?
                                                 PERSED

        Still at school   ☐

        Less than 3 full years at Secondary School   ☐

        3 or more years at Secondary School   ☐   PERFAMED

        Certified training course or apprenticeship   ☐

        University or Training College   ☐

   (b)   Do you have problems with learning or concentrating
      for long?
                       Yes ☐   No ☐   ☐

9.   Do you take part in any <u>clubs or groups</u>?
                                                CLUB
    (e.g. Sports, Social, Church)

                Yes ☐   No ☐

10.   Are you limited in any of the following activities
      compared with most people your age?

      (If you would not usually do the kind of activity in b) anyway,
      tick the end-box).

      a) PERSONAL NEEDS
         (bathing,toilet,dressing,eating)   Yes ☐   No ☐

      b) WORK ACTIVITIES AT HOME
         (Housework, cooking, gardening)   Yes ☐   No ☐   Don't ☐
                                                                do

      c) WORK OR EDUCATION TASKS
         (Concentration,ability to cope)   Yes ☐   No ☐

      d) GETTING ABOUT
         (Walking, stairs, recreations, in and Yes ☐   No ☐
         out of bed and vehicles)

      e) FINE AND SKILLED MOVEMENTS
         (Including ability to grip)   Yes ☐   No ☐

      f) COMMUNICATION
         (Speech, hearing, writing, reading)   Yes ☐   No ☐

      g) FITTING IN WITH SURROUNDINGS AND
         PEOPLE   Yes ☐   No ☐
         (Appreciation of time & space)
         (Quality of personal relationships)
         (Active interests, Enjoys events and outings)

11.   Do you usually have any trouble with:-

      Your eyes or seeing   Yes ☐   No ☐

      Your ears or hearing   Yes ☐   No ☐

      Mental Illness   Yes ☐   No ☐

      Getting about or moving   Yes ☐   No ☐
      parts of your body

      Any health problem or   Yes ☐   No ☐
      condition that is there
      all the time or keeps
      coming back.

      ┌───┐
      │   I N S T R U C T I O N S   │
      │ IF YOU ANSWERED 'YES' TO ANY OF THE ABOVE TICK BOX ☐ AND GO TO │
      │ Q 11.   │
      │ IF YOU ANSWERED 'NO' TO ALL THE ABOVE TICK BOX ☐ AND GO TO Q 16 │
      └───┘

12.   If you answered yes to any in Q 10 please describe below what
      is the trouble.

      ───

13(a) In general, when your trouble is present, <u>how much are you</u>
<u>limited</u> in what you want to do?

Not at all ☐   A little ☐   Quite a bit ☐   A lot ☐

(b) For how much of your time does it affect you?

Very little ☐   Little ☐   Quite a bit ☐   Most ☐   All ☐

DISLIM ☐

14.   Does your trouble or troubles cause <u>pain or discomfort</u>?

Yes ☐   No ☐

If yes:-

a) How much of your time does it worry you?

Very little ☐   Little ☐   Quite a bit ☐   Most ☐   All ☐

DISPAIN ☐

b) How <u>bad</u> is it usually?

Mild ☐   Moderate ☐   Severe ☐   Totally disabling ☐

c) Does this pain limit your abilities or enjoyment of life
(Taking into account the effectiveness of any pain relief)

Yes much ☐   Yes a little ☐   No ☐

15.   How <u>independent</u> are you and <u>how much help</u> do you need?
(Tick the box which describes your position best)

a) Independent and need no treatment and no help ☐

b) Independent, but need medicine or simple treatment ☐

DISDEP ☐

c) Independent, but have to make an extra effort to live
a full life. ☐

d) Independent, with the help of aids or appliances
(include mobility aids, catheters, hearing aids;
exclude glasses for reading or simple visual fault) ☐

e) Dependent on a helping hand at times ☐

f) Dependent on personal help to do things most of the
time. ☐

DISEV ☐

g) Dependent on help all of the time ☐

h) Completely dependent - bed nursing and help for all
activities ☐

— (i) Do you accept help (from equipment, medicine or people)
gladly when you need it.   Yes ☐   No ☐   ☐

— (j) Do you receive practical help and emotional support from

(a) family   Yes ☐   No ☐
(b) friends   Yes ☐   No ☐
(c) Community
services   Yes ☐   No ☐   N/A ☐   ☐

IN ANSWERING THE QUESTIONS ON THIS PAGE, PLEASE THINK
ONLY OF THE PAST 24 HOURS. MAKE NO ALLOWANCE FOR
INFORMATION YOU HAVE ALREADY GIVEN

16.   Have you had   any _illness_ or sign of _something wrong with your_
       health in the _last 24 hours_?

       (Including any caused by trouble you may have listed in Q 12)

                    Yes ☐   No ☐   ILLPREV

                                                                    ☐

                     I N S T R U C T I O N S

       IF YOU ANSWERED 'YES' TO THE ABOVE, TICK BOX ☐ AND GO TO Q 17

       IF YOU ANSWERED 'NO' TO THE ABOVE, TICK BOX ☐ AND GO TO Q 20

17.   If you answered 'yes' to Q 16 please explain briefly what was
       wrong with you.   ILLTYPE

       _____   ☐ 1

       _____   ☐ 2

       _____   ☐ 3

       _____   ☐ 4

18.   How has it affected what you could do over most of the last
       24 hours? (Tick one box)

   a) Felt well and could do the usual things for people my age ☐

   b) Felt unwell, but did my usual activities as well as usual ☐

   c) Not as efficient, but did usual activities. ☐

   d) Too unwell to do my usual activities but able to move   ILLSEV
      about at home ☐   ☐

   e) Confined to bed or couch but could do things for myself ☐

   f) Confined to bed and needing some help with washing,
      dressing or going to toilet. ☐

   g) Confined to bed and needed full nursing ☐

   h) Needed full bed nursing and not fully aware of
      surroundings ☐

   i) Unconscious ☐

19.   In general how are you feeling today?
       (may be answered by an observer in the household if necessary)

   a) Mentally
                  Enthusiastic ☐   ALERT
                  Bright and alert ☐   ☐
                  Rather subdued ☐
                  Withdrawn and unresponsive ☐
                  Unconscious ☐

   b) Physically
                                                    ACTIV
                  Exuberant ☐   ☐
                  Active ☐
                  Less active than usual ☐
                  Not getting about ☐   ALERT
                  Immobile in bed ☐   ☐

20. Have you ever had any <u>serious illness</u>, <u>accident</u> or <u>surgical operation</u>?
    (Include chronic illnesses such as asthma, diabetes, heart disease
    unless already noted in Q 11 and conditions requiring hospital
    admission or being off work for more than 1 week)

    Yes ☐   No ☐

HISTILL ☐

If yes	When	What

21. Do you have any real worries about

    (a) Health risks at work?   Yes ☐   No ☐

        If so, why_____

    (b) Your housing, because of size, condition or heating?
        Yes ☐   No ☐

    (c) Your diet - too little or unbalanced?   Yes ☐   No ☐

    (d) Other, environmental influences, eg. safe water
        supply or pollution?
        Yes ☐   No ☐

    (e) Your identity in the culture/society you live in?
        Yes ☐   No ☐

WORKRISK ☐

HOMRISK ☐

DIETRISK ☐

☐

☐

22. In the <u>last 12 months</u> have any of the following things happened to you?

    Death in the household or close family?   Yes ☐   No ☐

    Serious illness in the household or
    close family (including yourself)?   Yes ☐   No ☐

    Breakup with or serious worries about marital
    partner, close friend or close family members   Yes ☐   No ☐

    A change in where you live   Yes ☐   No ☐

    A change in your position or type of work   Yes ☐   No ☐

    A marked change in income   Yes ☐   No ☐

    Any other major change in your life   Yes ☐   No ☐

HISTRISK ☐

HISTRESS ☐

23. If an event like any of those in Q22 happened to you tomorrow do you think you would have good practical and emotional support from:

PRACS

family	Yes ☐	No ☐
friends	Yes ☐	No ☐
community services	Yes ☐	No ☐

☐

24   Here are some statements you could use to describe how you feel about yourself. Please read each statement carefully and place a tick in the column that fits you best. There are no right or wrong answers.

	Yes, that fits me exactly	Yes, that fits me more or less	That doesn't fit me either way.	No, that doesn't really fit me	No, that doesn't fit me at all.
a) If I really want to do things I can usually complete them					
b) I often find it difficult to cope with everyday problems					
c) I usually look forward to what each day will bring.					
d) I find it hard to relax and enjoy myself.					
e) I usually feel that I am a worthwhile person and that people value me.					
f) I tend to feel lonely or sad and anxious					
(g) I feel I can achieve worthwhile things.					
(h) I love others and am loved by others.					

☐ ☐ ☐ ☐ ☐ ☐ ☐ ☐

25.   How do you feel about the following?

ENJOY

☐

	Very happy	Happy	Fair	Not happy	Very disappointed
Home life					
Relations with family and friends					
Daily work or activities					
Social life/Recreation					
Financial Security					
Sex life					
Religion or philosophy					

26.   (a) Do you have : More good days than bad ☐   GOODBAD ☐

                      More bad days than good ☐

                      Couldn't say,most ordinary ☐

      (b) Can you say what thing, more than others, makes   GOODREAS ☐

          days - Good _____   BADREAS ☐

              Bad _____

27.   Below are some questions about everyday habits:-

      (a) Do you smoke?   Yes ☐   No ☐   SMOKE ☐

      (b) How much alcohol do you drink?   DRINK ☐

          None at all   ☐   Some, but less than 14 drinks ☐
                              a week on average
          Very occasional drink ☐   More than 14 drinks a week ☐
                                      on average

      (c) Do you usually get between 6½ - 8½ hours sleep a night? Yes ☐ No ☐   SLEEP ☐

      (d) Do you usually eat breakfast, lunch and dinner and   MEALS ☐
          little else in between?   Yes ☐ No ☐

      (e) Do you make a point of taking active exercise at   EXERCISE ☐
          least twice a week?   Yes ☐ No ☐

      (f) Please record:- your height_____your weight _____   WEIGHT ☐

          If height and weight not available, estimate If you are: WGTEST ☐

          Overweight ☐ About average ☐ Very underweight ☐

                                                            HELPRAC ☐

28.   Do you think you have a reasonable knowledge about the following:-
                                                Yes   No
      a) First aid and resuscitation   ☐   ☐   FIRSTAID ☐

      b) Child care   ☐   ☐   CHILD ☐

      c) Contraception and family planning   ☐   ☐   CONTRA ☐

      d) Sex   ☐   ☐   LOV ☐

      e) Nutrition and meal planning   ☐   ☐   NUTRIT ☐

      f) Checks for cancers and heart disease   ☐   ☐   CHECKS ☐

                                                            HELKNOW ☐

29. In the past year have you had:

(a) A dental check   Yes ☐   No ☐   SERVPREV

(b) A check of blood pressure   Yes ☐   No ☐   ☐
    (other than for its treatment)

(c) A screening check for cancer   Yes ☐   No ☐
    (e.g. breast or cervix)

(d) An injection to prevent disease   Yes ☐   No ☐
    (e.g. Tétanus, measles)

30. In the last month how many times have you seen a family doctor

or doctor at your place of work? If none write 0 _____   SEEDOC

                                                                        ☐

31. Do you feel confident that you can contact a doctor at short notice   DOCAVAIL

when you need one? Yes ☐   No ☐   Don't know ☐   ☐

32. Is there anyone other than a doctor who you can ask for advice when   ADVICE

someone in the house is first sick?   Yes ☐   No ☐   ☐

If yes, who is this person?   WHOAD

Family ☐ Neighbour or friend ☐ Chemist ☐ Infant or Public ☐   ☐
                                            Health Nurse

                                                        Other ☐

33. In the last month how many times have you been treated by any other kind

of health worker apart from a family doctor?   SEEOTHER

(e.g. Specialist, Accident and Emergency Staff, Community nurse,   ☐
  Physiotherapist, chiropractor, herbalist)

            If none write 0 _____

                                                                     WHOTHER
        If yes which type of health worker was it?_____

                                                                        ☐
34. In the last 12 months how many days have you spent as a hospital patient? SEEHOSP
            If none write 0 _____   ☐

                                                                     SERVCONT
                                                                        ☐
35. What is your opinion of your own health?   OWNFIT
     Very good ☐ Good ☐ Fair ☐ Poor ☐ Very Poor ☐   ☐

                                                                     HELSUP
                                                                        ☐

14
Functional Status Assessment in the Elderly

J. Heyrman, L. Dessers, M-B. De Munter, K. Haepers, and J. Craenen

The AMP Scoring System: An Instrument for Functional Status Evaluation of Elderly Patients

The AMP-scoring system was developed as part of a project for the production of an integrated computerized medical record for general practice (1). Its purpose is the assessment of functional status, primarily in the elderly, who are defined as persons aged 75 years and over. The assessment of functional status is particularly important in the elderly. Diagnostic assessments and decisions about therapeutic interventions require at least a possibility for improvements in health. The knowledge of functional status as a measurement of health is very important.

The AMP system was designed as one of several registration instruments with the expectation that functional status assessment would expand the clinical horizons of the general practitioner.

A literature search failed to reveal an assessment instrument that was practical for use by general practitioners. Some were too complicated and others were too limited in scope. The AMP instrument assesses global function in three areas, each with three components. Severity is rated on a scale of from 1 to 4 as follows:

1. There is no problem.
2. Small problems exist, but function is not impaired.
3. The patient requires help in this area.
4. There is serious impairment.

Physicians are asked to score each area of function (AMP) as follows:
  A means Activity, where

a is an assessment of *activities* of daily living,

b refers to how *busy* the person is, for example, the extended activities of daily living, and

c refers to *condition*, such as vision, hearing, and walking.

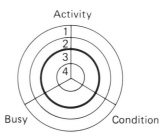

M means mental status, where

m is *memory* function,
n is *normal care* of possessions, and
o means *orientation* in time and space.

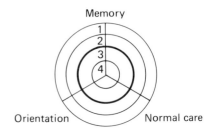

Memory

P means psychosocial status, where

p refers to ability to rational *plans*,
r indicates *relationships* with important persons, and
s indicates *social supports*.

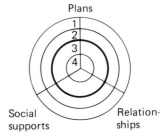

Plans

Scoring is linked to the notion of autonomy versus dependency. Patients who score either 1 or 2 are generally autonomous, whereas a score of 3 indicates passage into dependency. The circle separating score 2 from score 3 is therefore drawn thicker than the other circles. A score of 4 indicates a considerable amount of dependency.

The AMP scoring system has several advantages. It is designed to be completed by the physician, not by the patient. It is expected that the information recorded will be useful for both diagnostic and therapeutic decisions. The assessment is global and includes activities of daily living and other aspects of function. Yet there are only nine items that require assessment. The focus is on the seriousness of the problem rather than on actual performance measurements. The assessments are therefore more likely to help the physician decide whether action is needed.

Other advantages include the mnemonic aids and the visual overview as noted in the illustrations below. Physicians can quickly determine which functional areas are impaired and plan for interventions in the hope of improving the patient's health status.

A means activity, where

a is an assessment of *activities* of daily living,
b refers to how *busy* the person is: the extended activities of daily living,
c refers to body *condition* such as vision, hearing, walking.

The AMP Scoring System

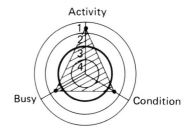

Activity

1. no problem
2. small problems, satisfactory functioning
3. without help not possible
4. serious problems

M means mental status, where
m *memory* function;
n *normal care* of possessions, and
o *orientation* in time and space.

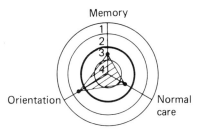

Memory

Orientation

Normal care

1. no problem
2. small problems, satisfactory functioning
3. without help, not possible
4. lack off good mental functioning, serious problems

P means psychosocial status; where
p refers to ability to make rational *plans*,
r indicates *relationships* with important persons, and
s *social supports*.

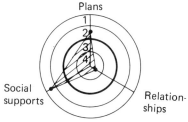

Plans

Social supports

Relationships

1. no problems
2. small problems, satisfactory functioning
3. problems, more social support necessary
4. lack of good psychosocial adjustment, serious problems

Field Trial Results

A field trial with the AMP instrument was preceded by a study of the attitudes and opinions about functional status assessment of 15 general practitioners who were asked to assess, in a free-text form, patients aged 75 years and over (624 registrations in three months of recording). Of the "free-text" assessments, 50% included only one statement, mostly on activities of daily living; another 25% included two statements, and in no case were more than four aspects of functional status written down. Only 15% of the assessments included psychosocial components. For this preliminary phase, we constructed an autonomy score for elderly patients using the technique of content analysis of the free-text statements described by Holst (2). On this basis (3), 30% of the contacts were classified as autonomous, 2% as semidependent, and 18% as very dependent. We were unable to classify the other 50% because of the lack of useful information.

For the field trial, 9 general practitioners out of the previous 15 assessed 302 patients aged 75 and over during a three-month period using the AMP system and scoring all nine components of function on a scale of seriousness of from 1 to 4. Here 30% of the patients were classified as autonomous, 35% as semidependent (with a score of three in at least one axis), and 35% as very dependent (with a score of four in at least one axis). Comparing the free text assessment to the structured AMP assessment, the AMP scoring system seems to help the GP in classifying the group of 50% uncertain patients he left out in the free text score. The group labelled as semi-dependent increased from 2% to 35%, which is extremely important, because this is the borderline group where actions have to focus on.

The physicians retained a copy of the AMP charts in their patient's records, and six months later they were interviewed on the usefulness of the instrument. They felt that the instrument had broadened their scope of patient assessment, that it had given valuable and constantly available information, and that it had provided insight into changes over time. The visual pattern representation was considered superior to aggregate or individual scores. Most physicians felt that it should be an integral part of the basic medical record.

In summary, the AMP scoring system is a useful, interesting instrument for assessing the functional status of elderly patients. Its validity requires additional testing.

References

1. Heyrman J, Dessers L: Development of instruments for computerization of an integrated medical record for general practice. NFWO-grant 3/9005/87/N.
2. Holst OR: Content Analysis. In: Lindzey G and Aroson E. *The Handbook of Social Psychology.* London: Addison-Wesley; 1968:601.
3. De Munter B: *The General Practitioner and the Elderly in Primary Care, an Explorative Study on the Registration Behavior of 14 GP's.* Leuven, Belgium: Catholic University of Leuven; 1988. Thesis.

A Scoring System for Family Coping

The family coping scoring system was developed as part of a research project for the production of an integrated computerized medical record in general practice. A medical record is not only an instrument for the bookkeeping of facts, it is also a basic structure for handling medical reality. Which facts are the most interesting to collect, and which framework structures reality in the most convenient way?

Theoretical Background

In recent years, research focusing on the relationship between environmental factors and health has emphasized that the susceptibility to and the course of diseases is strongly influenced by the way people deal with stressors in their environment (1–6).

FAMILY COPING

People's reactions to these stressful events have been consolidated in the concept of "coping behavior." A considerable amount of coping literature confirms the assumption that the way people react to burdensome events has important repercussions on their physical, psychological, and social well-being (1, 7–10). Environmental factors, including family relationships, may transform an innocuous relationship between the agent of disease and the individual into clinical disease. Therefore, we need to examine family and environmental factors that alter or change the relationship between the individual and these ubiquitous agents of disease (11).

When disease can be seen as a result of inefficient coping with certain stressors in the environment, it can also be a stressful event itself, for which coping mechanisms need to be developed. Depending on the stage and the severity of the illness, the whole social system surrounding the patient will be afflicted, and become involved. Besides coping with the disease, people must also learn to cope with the diseased individual as a person. The course of a disease is often strongly influenced by the interaction between the ill person and his/her environment, and in the first place, his or her family. Here also, a system (family) approach will be the most appropriate way to help the patient. Briefly, coping with disease is not an individual but a family affair, that is, "family coping" (12).

Why is it that some families are better "copers" than other families, who face similar if not identical stressors or family transitions? This remains the major question in family stress research (13).

FAMILY TYPOLOGY

Family stress theory assumes that certain family "types" play a buffering role with respect to stressful events, and thus facilitate family adaptation (14). Many researchers have developed family assessment measures to examine and test the strengths and shortcomings of this assumption (15–23). "The use of family assessment measures in health care research and practice is based upon the premise that family functioning interacts with individual physiological and psychological processes in a discernable and predictable manner, and consequently affects the health status of the family members" (p. 53) (24). These pattern of family functioning are reinforced by rules and norms and guided by family values and goals. As soon as these characteristics can be identified and measured, it is possible to classify each family or place it within a typology. Furthermore, these typologies can be used to make predictions about how a particular family may react when faced with stressful life circumstances (24). Briefly, these family typologies leads us to better understand the durability and capability of families in the face of an ever-changing social situation.

FAMILY COHESION

Most of the family typologies consist of pairs of family variables instead of a single family dimension. Two of the major variables, which most of these typologies have in common, are linked to cohesion and adaptability. Cohesion refers to the emotional bonding between family members. The terms *togetherness* (25) and *bonding* (26) are sometimes used in the same sense. *Adaptability* is defined as the ability of a family system to change its power structure, role relationships, and relationship rules in response to situational and developmental stress (19, 21, 22). The term *flexibility* (20, 26) has a similar meaning.

PERSONALITY STRENGTH

Researching in a global way the question of who is getting diseased and who stays in "health-ease," personality characteristics are important. In 1979, Antonowsky (1) developed the concept of *the sense of coherence*, defined as the pervasive feeling of confidence in the predictability of internal and external environments. It proves the most powerful dimension of general resistance to disease (2).

THE DOCTOR IN RELATION TO THE FAMILY

Depending on the type of family the general practitioner is facing, the roles and expectations attributed to him may differ considerably. According to Haley (27), helping professionals should be included in the conceptualization of any therapeutic treatment system with a family, since family structure and functioning play a part in understanding and managing the complaint of the individual patient as well as of the family in trouble. Smilkstein (22) focused upon the family unit as part of "medical" care and treatment. In medicine, this idea has led to various forms of "The Therapeutic Triangle" (28). This triangle includes the patient, the family, and the physician.

The Family Scoring System Project

In the project, an attempt was made to operationalize this integrated approach for application in the general practitioner's office. We integrated different aspects of family coping into a single diagram. We selected personality strength as the x-axis and family cohesion as the y-axis. Three concentric circles represent the severity of the problem, as follows:

1. essentially no problem
2. a problem exists, but the patient copes well
3. a serious problem

For reasons of clarity, we tried to coordinate the four doctor–family relationship typologies with family typology. The four quadrants of personality strength and family cohesion demonstrate a relational typology, as follows:

A. *Doctor as a friend*, the family has good cohesion and the patient has a strong personality.

B. *Doctor as a competitor*, the patient has a strong personality, but the family has poor cohesion.

C. *Doctor as a godfather*, the family has good cohesion, but the patient's personality is weak.

D. *Doctor as a threat*, the patient has a weak personality and the family has poor cohesion. (See the figure below.)

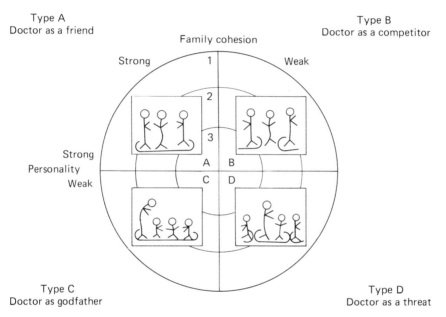

1) Essentially no problem
2) A problem exists but the patient copes well
3) A serious problem

We asked the physicians to define their relationship with the family using the above typology, since we thought that the doctor's concept of how the family system defines his or her role might provide useful information. The diagram is constructed in a fashion similar to that of the AMP scoring system and we attempted to combine the three major areas into a single score.

FIELD SCORE

Nine physicians were asked to score patients aged 75 and over and their coping strengths; 302 patients were assessed, and a copy of the diagram was put each patients' medical record. Six months later, the doctors were interviewed concerning the usefulness of the instrument.

TABLE 14.1. Frequency distribution of doctor typology scores in relation to elderly patients ($N = 377$) and their families.

Doctor typology	N	Percent
A, Doctor as friend	249	66.0
B, Doctor as competitor	22	5.8
C, Doctor as godfather	91	24.1
D, Doctor as threat	15	4.0

Scoring their relationship with patients was difficult for the doctors because it required an assessment of their own behavior and of their wish for certain types of relationships with the families of the patients they were treating. Some physicians realized that they always wished to be regarded as a friend, whereas different patterns emerged for other physicians (Table 14.1).

The field test provided interesting insights into physician–patient relationships although additional research is required to establish the usefulness of the coping instrument and its relationship to functional assessment.

Acknowledgment. This research project was granted by the Belgian government. NFWO-grant 3/9005/87/N.

References

1. Antonovsky A: *Health, Stress, and Coping: New Perspectives on Mental and Physical Well-Being.* San Francisco, Jossey-Bass, 1979.
2. Antonovsky A: *Unraveling the Mystery of Health: How People Manage Stress and Stay Well.* San Francisco, Jossey-Bass, 1979.
3. Dohrenwend BS, Dohrenwend BP: *Stressful Life Events: Their Nature and Effects.* New York, Wiley 1974.
4. Dohrenwend BP, Dohrenwend BS (eds): *Stressful Life Events and Their Contexts. Series in Psychological Epidemiology, Nr. 2,* New Brunswick, NJ, Rutgers University Press, 1981.
5. Fisher S, Reason J (eds): *Handbook of Life Stress, Cognition and Health.* New York, Wiley, 1988.
6. Kaplan HB (ed): *Psychosocial Stress: Trends in Theory and Research.* New York, Academic Press, 1983.
7. Coelho GV, Hamburg DA, Adams JE: *Coping Adaptation.* New York, Basic Books, 1974.
8. Cohen F, Lazarus RS: *Coping with the Stress of illness,* in Stone GC, Cohen, F Adler NE (eds): *Health Psychology: A Handbook.* San Francisco, Jossey-Bass, 1979.
9. Pearlin L, Schooler C: The structure of coping. *J Health Soc Behav* 19:2–21, 1978.
10. Ursin H: Activation, coping, and psychosomatics, in Ursin H, Baade E, Levine S (eds): *Psychobiology of Stress: A Study of Coping Men.* New York, Academic Press, 1978.
11. Cassel J: The contribution of the social environment to host resistance. *Am J Epidemiol* 104:107–123, 1976.

12. McCubbin HI, McCubbin MA, Patterson JM, Cauble AE, Wilson LR, Warwick W: Coping health inventory for patients: an assessment of parential coping patterns in the care of the chronically III child. *J Marriage and the Fam* 45:359–371, 1983.

13. McCubbin HI, McCubbin MA: Family stress theory and assessment: The T-double ABCX model of family adjustment and adaptation, in McCubbin HI, Thompson AI (eds): *Family Assessment Inventories for Research and Practice.* Madison, University of Wisconsin, pp. 3–34, 1987.

14. McCubbin HI, Thompson AI, Pirner P: *Family Rituals Typologies and Family Strengths. Family Stress Coping and Health Project,* Madison, University of Wisconsin, 1986.

15. Epstein N, Bishop D, Baldwin L: McMaster model of family functioning: A view of the normal family, in Walsh F (ed): *Normal Family Processes.* New York, Guilford Press, 1982.

16. Epstein N, Levin S, Bishop D: The family as a social unit. *Can Fam Phys* 22:1411–1413, 1976.

17. McCubbin HI, Thompson AI (eds): *Family Assessment Inventories for Research and Practice.* Madison, University of Wisconsin, 1987.

18. Moos RH: *Family Environment Scales.* Palo Alto, CA, Consulting Psychologists Press, 1974.

19. Olson DH, Portner J, Bell R: *Family Adaptability and Cohesion Evaluation Scales. Family Social Science.* St. Paul, University of Minnesota, 1978.

20. Olson DH, Portner J, Bell R: *FACES II: Family Adaptability and Cohesion Evaluation Scales. Family Social Science.* St. Paul, University of Minnesota, 1982.

21. Olson DH, Portner J, Lavee Y: *FACES III: Family Adaptability and Cohesion Evaluation Scales. Family Social Science.* St. Paul, University of Minnesota, 1985.

22. Smilkstein G: The family APGAR: A proposal for a family function test and its use by physicians. *J Fam Prac* 6:1231–1239, 1978.

23. Steinhauer PS, Santa Barbara J, Skinner HA: The process model of family functioning. *Can J Psychiat* 29:77–88, 1984.

24. McCubbin HI, McCubbin MA: Family system assessment in health care, in McCubbin HI, Thompson AI (eds): *Family Assessment Inventories for Research and Practice.* Madison, University of Wisconsin, pp. 52–78, 1987.

25. McCubbin HI, McCubbin MA, Thompson AI: Family time and routines scale, in McCubbin HI, Thompson AI (eds): *Family Assessment Inventories for Research and Practice.* Madison, University of Wisconsin, pp. 133–144, 1987.

26. McCubbin HI, Olson DH, Lavee Y, Patterson JM: Family index of resiliency and adaptation, in McCubbin HI, Thompson AI (eds): *Family Assessment Inventories for Research and Practice.* Madison, University of Winconsin, pp. 285–305, 1987.

27. Haley J: *Problem-Solving Therapy.* San Francisco, Jossey-Bass, 1976.

28. Doherty, WJ, Baird MA: *Family Therapy and Family Medicine: Toward the Primary Care of Families.* New York, Guilford Press, 1983.

15
Studies Using the Nottingham Health Profile in General Practice

C. VAN WEEL, A.J.A. SMITS, and W.J.H.M. VAN DEN BOSCH

Introduction

Patients present complaints or problems to the (family) doctor. After assessing the problem the doctor intervenes. Usually, the patient is sent on his way and will only come back for the same problem in the case of insufficient response to his treatment. This is particularly true for an acute, less serious illness such those that are predominantly treated in primary care. The monitoring of outcome is mainly implicit and rests with the patient. If he is satisfied with the final result, he does not return to the practice. Medical follow-up is by and large restricted to cases in which there is a discrepancy between expected and experienced outcome.

There are several developments in primary care that question the limitations of this implicit but pragmatic way of assessing outcome of care. These include

a growing emphasis on chronic morbidity;
a growing emphasis on prevention and asymptomatic conditions; and
a growing emphasis on research.

The question then is: What outcome is to be measured? This is not easy to answer; much depends on whether the treatment has effected a change in health status. Also health in itself is a hybrid concept.

Health Status

Health is defined as "the state of complete somatic, social and psychic well-being, and not the mere absence of illness" (1). One of the implications of this ambiguous definition is the impossibility of approaching health by one measure or scale. It can be deduced that the following aspects are part of the concept:

somatic status
psychosocial status; and
socioeconomic status.

The three aspects are in themselves broad and diverse. Even more important is the interrelationships between them. The definition stongly suggests equal parity. But how does a disturbance in social status compare with a physical impairement? For the time being, it is sensible to restrict measurement to bits and pieces, without too much worry whether it can be seen as a true index of "health."

Subjective Health Assessment

The problem of assessing health is further complicated by the question of who is to be the assessor. The above description of the current implicit practice points to an essetial role of the patient in this proces. Common sense will support this, since the ulimate aim of medical care is to promote and reinforce patients' health. Should a patient judge his condition after a medical intervention as unsatisfactory, then there is sufficient reason to question effectiveness of the intervention.

It must be stressed, however, that the motives to seek a more objective scale of outcome are in part physician centered. The effect of intervention in preventive care and the treatment of mild, asymptomatic, and chronic diseases need careful supervision in the monitoring of the quality of care. The patients' (subjective) assessment of his health is only a part and probably a minor part of the relevant data in this respect.

The Nottingham health profile (NHP) is a tool to measure perceived health. Our experience with this instrument will be described, with particular emphasis on

the relationships with other health/morbidity indicators;
relevance in the clinical context; and
the sensitivity to changes in health/morbidity.

The Nottingham Health Profile

The NHP is a list of 45 questions, phrased to be answered in a simple yes/no way (2). The questions can be reduced to the following six dimensions:

energy;
pain;
emotional reactions;
sleep;
social isolation; and
physical mobility.

The score (a weighted sum score) has a range of 0 to 100 (3). The nonprofessional system has been used to develop the scoring system. Normal values for sex and age are available (3).

The NHP was developed in the United Kingdom. It has been possible to translate the list into Dutch without loss of reliability and validity; there are no indications of transcultural problems (4). Subgroups of different age, sex, and medical history show different profiles in scores.

The Nottingham Health Profile and Old Patients

The NHP was used in a study to analyze the health and medical needs of very old patients of a health center in Eindhoven, The Netherlands (5). The aim of this study was to assess the hidden needs of patients 75 years old and older so that a preventive program could be planned. All the patients in this age group on the practice list were allocated to one of two groups, according to their consumption of medical services: (i) a group of regular attenders of primary care: all patients with at least two contacts with either the family physician or the district nurse in the year preceding the study and (ii) a group of non-attenders of primary care: patients who had not seen either the family physician or the district nurse in the year preceding the study.

A sample of 50 patients in each subgroup was studied. The following information was collected:

1. Morbidity (overt and hidden); a history was taken and a physical examination was performed, with special attention to chronic diseases (6). The medical record was checked to see whether the conditions discovered had already been identified in primary care.
2. Activities of daily life (ADL) (7).
3. NHP scores.

None of the patients was institutionalized. All patients had to provide their own support. Among the nonattenders there were more males and more couples living together than there were among the attenders. Very old patients were found more often in the attenders' group.

All the information gathered was presented to the family physician, without instructions for follow-up or intervention. Actions taken by the family doctor, however, were recorded. The interpretation of information by the family physician in terms of interventions or follow-ups is further referred to as "the clinical context."

Morbidity, Daily Life Performance, and the Nottingham Health Profile

The medical examination revealed an impressive number of signs or symptoms of chronic conditions (Table 15.1): 74 among the attenders and 60 among the nonattenders. The greatest number was among the nonattenders; here 40 new potential conditions were detected, compared to 24 among the attenders.

The mobility of the two groups appeared to be good (Table 15.2): Most of the patients were able to perform essential daily activities without the need of support from others. The NHP scores are summarized in Table 15.3. On average, male patients reported fewer symptoms or problems or both than female patients. There were no important differences between the attenders

TABLE 15.1. Patients with signs–symptoms of chronic morbidity.

	Number of patients with signs–symptoms	
Condition	Attenders[a]	Nonattenders[a]
Chronic obstructive lung disease	6 (1)	8 (7)
Heart failure	4 (0)	6 (5)
Angina pectoris	5 (2)	7 (5)
Prostate hypertrophy	3 (2)	0
Incontinence	11 (7)	8 (8)
Arthritis	10 (1)	9 (9)
Deafness	20 (8)	4 (4)
Impaired vision	9 (0)	11 (0)
Anemia	1 (1)	2 (2)
Hypertension	2 (0)	1 (0)
Dementia	3 (2)	4 (0)
Total	74 (24)	60 (40)

[a]The numbers in parentheses are the number of patients with previously unknown signs–symptoms.

TABLE 15.2. Activities of daily living.

Number of impaired functions	Attenders	Nonattenders
0	41	44
1	5	3
2	2	1
3	1	2
4	2	0
5–8	0	0
Total	51	50

TABLE 15.3. Average score of the Nottingham Health Profile.

NHP dimension	Attenders male/female	Nonattenders male/female	Standard 75+ male/female
Energy	6.2/10.7	14.6/20.3	29.3/44.0
Pain	8.6/ 6.1	6.1/11.5	14.1/25.9
Sleep	9.3/18.6	4.4/ 9.7	30.6/29.9
Emotions	8.8/ 8.1	13.4/16.6	12.8/16.6
Social isolation	18.1/11.7	5.7/14.2	9.8/12.1
Mobility	10.9/21.9	9.5/16.6	21.3/36.1

and the nonattenders. Both groups had a lower score than the (sex- and age-specific) standard score.

The correlation of morbidity, ADL performance, and NHP score did show that patients with the highest number of signs and symptoms and chronic morbidity had the highest NHP scores. Patients reporting impaired daily life activities also had the highest NHP scores. High and low NHP scores, however, could not be explained by either chronic morbidity or daily life activities impairment.

The Health Assessment

The study described here aimed to assess the health status of old patients in primary care. The data were interpreted in their "clinical" context: the possibility of hidden morbidity, unmet needs, and *dis*-functioning with the potential of intervention. Their interpretation led to the following conclusions:

1. Screening by medical examination did disclose a number of previously unindentified chronic health problems. Follow-up led to only a few interventions: 12 cases (fewer than 20% of all identified cases), mainly for visual and hearing aids. There may be some impact on the quality of life, but the impact on future morbidity seemed to be limited. The cost-effectiveness of this method of screening was low (8).

2. The assessment of ADL performance contained the most information. It directly modified the discovery of chronic morbidity. The cases of arthritis, chronic obstructive pulmonary disease, and heart failure could be related to its impact on daily life. Limitations in therapeutic interventions were mainly based on knowledge of the conditions' limited consequences for daily activities.

Information on the ability to perform activities of everyday life were of direct relevance as well. The discovery of an impairment in this respect required follow-up to provide support if needed. The overall yield, however, was limited, since all patients were receiving support for impaired functions; in the case of the nonattenders, this support had apparently been arranged through the initiative of nonprofessionals (i.e., laymen).

3. The NHP scores did correlate in part with the findings of the other two instruments, notably, the ADL performance scale. This can be explained by similarities between the questionnaires: the NHP contains a number of questions more or less identical with the ADL scale. However, some patients reported high levels of perceived health problems without apparent chronic morbidity or impaired ADL (6). The NHP measures aspects of health in its own right, aspects that are not covered by other approaches. This is in line with the previous experience in the validation of the original NHP (2) or its translated version (4). Our experience with the group of very old patients in primary care, however, revealed that the additional information from the NHP was not very useful in the clinical context. The aim of the survey was to plan for individual preventive action on the basis of information about hidden

needs. The overall (group level) NHP information did indicate satisfactory levels of perceived health. As a consequence, the need for interventions was limited. The ADL performance scale was clinically more informative. The NHP score alone did not lead to any follow-up action or intervention for any individual patient in this survey.

The Nottingham Health Profile and Young Adults

In this study 120 young adults (age 30 to 40 years) took part. The aim of the project was to study the prognosis of early childhood morbidity. The 120 patients belong to the practice population of one of the four practices of the Continuous Morbidity Registration Nijmegen (6, 9). They formed the total group on the practice list in 1988, and had been listed with the same practice for 20–40 years. Their childhood morbidity was recorded and analyzed over the years 1945–1965 in a study on family patterns in morbidity (10). The complete medical life history of these patients is available (E-list) (9, 11).

All patients have been screened for the most prevalent (presymptomatic) diseases of childhood and adulthood (6).

The screening consisted of a standard history, a physical examination, and a laboratory work-up. All the patients completed an NHP. Only the first crude data of this study are available so far; the NHP scores and a global relation of NHP score to early childhood morbidity is presented. The physical screening did not reveal important chronic or severe illness in the study group.

Nottingham Health Profile Scores

The NHP scores are given in Table 15.4. The majority of patients did not report any perceived health problems (range: 76% for emotion; 96% for mobility). High scores are the exception. This is in line with common experience: Psychosocial problems are prevalent in this age group, but painful, immobilization conditions are rare.

The Nottingham Health Profile and Childhood Morbidity

Table 15.5 relates the NHP scores to global parameters of morbidity in childhood. The greater the number of episodes of illness as a child, the higher

TABLE 15.4. The Nottingham Health Profile score (percentage) of 120 adults.

NHP score	Energy	Emotion	Pain	Sleep	Mobility	Isolation
0	93	76	91	85	96	89
1 to 29	3	20	7	12	4	8
30 to 100	4	4	2	3	0	3

TABLE 15.5. Adult NHP score and early childhood morbidity.

Characteristics of early childhood morbidity		NHP score at adulthood
Number of episodes	<7	9.5
	≥7	18
Severe episodes	<3	11
	≥3	19
Not severe episodes	<5	8
	≥5	21

the NHP score. This is also true for the number of serious and nonserious illness episodes.

The Health Assessment of Young Adults

The NHP scores seem to be related to the medical history—in this case, to the level of childhood morbidity. It is the presentation of morbidity to the family physician rather than the severity of these childhood episodes that determines this relationship.

However, the pattern is havily influenced by a few patients with very high NHP scores. It is the authors' impression that manifest psychosocial morbidity will be the major factor in the health profile of these patients. This is part of the current analysis in the study.

This hypothetical explanation of this finding is in line with analysis of psychosocial (14) or nervous–functional complaints in primary care: psychosocial problems do form the single most important factor in determining the use of medical facilities. In the study population there was a clear family trait in presenting health problems in primary care (10, 13). This could be demonstrated up to the third generation.

Conclusions and Recommendations

The NHP is introduced as a new tool for clinicians and epidemiologists (2). It assesses perceived health on the basis of a list of 45, simple-to-answer questions. The score has been subdivided into six dimensions: energy, pain, emotions, sleep, social isolation, and physical mobility. The instrument makes a contribution of its own in approximating health (3, 4). The instrument is validated (3, 4), and it has been possible to translate and adapt the list into Dutch without a loss of its test capacities (5).

The scores relate on aggregate to basic health characteristics of groups: old patients (65 +) and women are known to have a different health status than younger adults and men, and these groups show a higher NHP score; patients with a chronic disease also score more symptoms/health problems (5).

The NHP is claimed to be of clinical value as well. Its clinical aspects were tested in a study of the health status of very old patients. Two major problems in this respect were noted:

1. the overlap with shorter assessment tools, that is, the ADL performance scale;
2. the lack of individual implications in the provision of health care following scoring of NHP profiles.

Redundancy of information has been reported by others (14). It points to methodological problems in NHP testing. The fact is, family doctors can interpret a functional assessment like the assessment of ADL performance much better. The redundancy problem can be underscored in the survey among the very old patients: the question of how people assessed their own health was directly related to high or low NHP scores. The validation of the NHP did use lay assessments (5), so this finding is probably not surprising. Whatever the potential of clinical interpretation of this type of patient's subjective qualification, it is more cost-effective to answer this single question than a set of 45 questions. An additional problem of the NHP has been reported: Indicators of health should be sensitive to change in health status. So far there is little experience with this aspect, but there is sufficient ground to doubt the NHP in this respect (14).

Perceived health assessment is of special importance when other assessment strategies can be expected to achieve little. The experience with young adults can be helpful here. The use of health status indicators in this study was more research-oriented and less clinical than in the study of very old patients.

This aspect of clinical interpretation has not been followed up in depth, but the experience can nevertheless be used to estimate the value of NHP. There were important differences in NHP scores between "healthy" adults; an extreme number of perceived health problems in a few individuals determined the distribution of the scores. Also the NHP measured an aspect of health overlooked in the "traditional" surveillance by medical history and physical examination. The current perceived health relates in some way to the number of illness episodes presented to the family physician in childhood.

Use of medical facilities is largely determined by psychosocial problems, problem behavior, or nervous–functional complaints(14); on a family scale, these patterns of use of health facilities strongly predict consultation frequency in (early) childhood. There are indications in the group of patients studied here, that psychosocial problems are the (or a) primary explanation of the NHP scores. if this is the case, perceived health is mainly determined by psychosocial morbidity. The use of NHP as an outcome measure in the clinical sense will, under those conditions, be limited: Thus, there are simpler ways to assess this aspect in individuals and groups of patients and the NHP can be expected to be a stable characteristic of patients, rather than sensitive to change (12), since chronic problem behavior or nervous–functional complaints are a lasting characteristic of patients.

Summing Up

The experiences in the two studies described here, confirm the fact that the NHP measures specific aspects of health status. Perceived health is a distinct part of health status, and at least in part independent of other aspects. NHP can be measured reliably, and without many problems can be adapted for different "cultures."

Our experience casts doubt on the clinical use in assessing of the NHP health status as an outcome of episodes of illness. The complexity of the instrument, the broad aspects of health it attempts to cover, and the abstract way of summarizing the results can be held responsible for this.

The experiences described here point to the potential of assessment of function in this respect. The simple terms in which function can be measured allows for direct medical interpretation from the identified impaired functions. The NHP appears to be the instrument of epidemiologists and sociomedical researchers. Family physicians and other clinicians should turn to the assessment of function and the change of functional capacity as their most relevant indicator of outcome of illness and therapy.

References

1. World Health Organization. Constitution of the World Health Organization, In *Basic Documents*. Geneva, World Health Organization, p. 2, 1948.
2. Hunt SM, McEwen J, McKenna SP: Measuring health status: A new tool for clinicians and epidemiologists. *J R Coll Gen Pract* 35:185–188, 1985.
3. McEwen J: Manual: *The Nottingham Health Profile*. London, Academic Department of Community Medicine, 1985.
4. Eyk JTM, Smits AJA, Meyboom W, Mokkink H, Son J van: The Nottingham Health Profile in the Dutch situation. *Allgemeinmedizin* (accepted for publication).
5. Weel C van, Thissen E, Kock Th, Klaassen J, Felix W, Gooskens P, Wosten P: Preventive care for the elderly. *Allgemeinmedizin* 18:70–73, 1989.
6. Hoogen HJM, Huygen FJA, Schellekens JWG, Straat J, Velden HGM van der: *Morbidity Figures from General Practice*. Department of Family Medicine, University of Nijmegen, Nijmegen, The Netherlands, 1985.
7. Katz S, Branch LG, Banson MH, Papsidero JA, Beck JC, Greer DS: Active life expectancy. *N Engl J Med* 309:1218–1224, 1983.
8. Williams EL: Scope for intervention following case identification, In Taylor RC, Buckley EG, (eds): *Preventive Care for the Elderly*. Occasional Paper 35, London, Royal College of General Practitioners, 1987.
9. Weel C van, Bosch WJHM van den, Hoogen HJM van den, Smits AJA: Development of respiratory illness in childhood—a longitudial study in general practice. *J R Coll Gen Pract* 37:404–408, 1987.
10. Huygen FJA: *Family Medicine, the Medical Life History of Families*. Nijmegen, The Netherlands, Dekker en van der Vegt, 1978.
11. College of General Practitioners: A classification of disease. *J R Coll Gen Pract* 2:140–159, 1959.

12. Kind P, Carr-Hill R: The Nottingham Health profile: A useful tool for epidemio logists? *Soc Sci Med* 25:905–910, 1987.
13. Huygen FJA: Longitudinal studies of family units. *J R Coll Gen Pract.* 38:170, 1988.
14. Lamberts H: Problem behavior in primary health care. *J R Coll Gen Pract* 29:331–335, 1979.

16
Position Paper on the Assessment of Functional Status in Primary Care in a Developing Country—Pakistan

M.H. MIRZA

Primary care in a developing country differs markedly from a similar level of care in fully developed countries. Instruments designed to assess functional status in use in developed countries, therefore, require modification if they are to be incorporated into the daily practice of Pakistani family physicians.

The WHO definition of health as "a state of complete physical, mental, and social well-being, and not merely the absence of disease or infirmity" is even less useful for developing countries than it is for those countries that are more developed. The ability of family physicians in primary care settings to assess their patients' health requires a full knowledge of their cultural and spiritual backgrounds. Quantification of these variables as components of health status is very difficult.

Additional difficulties are encountered with the assessment of patients' presenting complaints. Important information may be suppressed or presented in an ambiguous fashion, thus masking the patients' true psychosocial status. Seemingly adequate social support may have negative components or adverse consequences on the health of the patient. Patients' spiritual belief may also modify the presentation of symptoms and interfere with a full assessment of health and disease.

Is the assessment of pain during the preceding 4 weeks a correct measure of functional status? Painful menstruation (dysmenorrhea) occurring monthly is often considered a normal phenomenon and may or may not modify the woman's functional status.

The assessment of daily work between the extremes of fully satisfied to dissatisfied with a monotonous and repetitive job is affected by more than the person's physical and emotional states. Are there coexisting social problems such as uncooperative colleagues in teamwork?

Assessment of quality of life presents additional difficulties. Is a person in an underdeveloped or developing country assessing quality of life in relationship to people and conditions in his or her own country or relative to living conditions in fully developed countries? My preference is that quality of life be defined as "a state of normalcy in physical and mental terms and complete

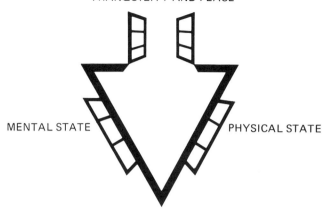

FIGURE 16.1. The three-dimensional concept is illustrated wherein the physical state and mental state have their outlet through quality of life into a world of peace and tranquility.

harmony with the environment at a particular point in time and for a period of time."

Considering the above comments, I would suggest a three-dimensional instruments that measures physical, mental, and quality of life components of functional status in terms of optimal states as related to relevant groups. The optimal functional status is determined through the straight alignment of the windows of an ideal cluster opening to the door of tranquility and satisfaction in an environment of serenity and peace (Figure 16.1).

The instrument (Figure 16.2) could be either self-administered on administered by paramedical or research people. Patients should rate their status on the several scales, which scores should be verified by the doctor.

Some clusters such as social status are interdependent and complementary to others. Taken together these ratings could indicate optimal status such as "feeling on top of the world" as an assessment of quality of life. The model appears appropriate for use by family physicians and has been useful in my own office setting. Additional testing to assess reliability and validity, however, is required.

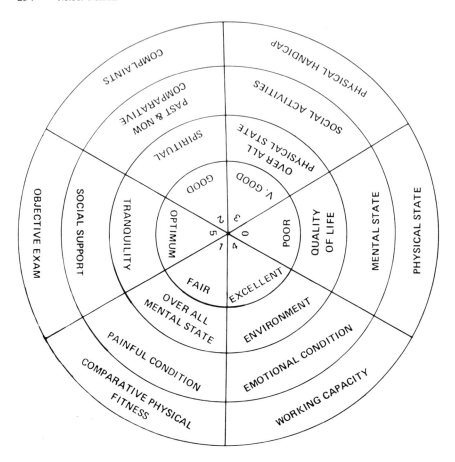

FIGURE 16.2. For spinwheel use, a number from 0 to 5 (optimum) is brought into alignment with a component of the desired parameter, namely, physical state, mental state, and quality of life depending on the quantifier, namely, poor, fair, good, and very good.

The spinwheel scorecard assesses the different parameters under physical state from 0 to 5 (optimum). Mental state and quality of life parameters are accordingly assessed and are quantified on the scorecard.

Scorecard Assessment of functional status in a primáry care setting in the developing country Pakistan.

Patient's Name————————————————————
Date of Birth———————————— Sex: Male————————
                                  Female————————

Spinwheel	Score
Physical state	Optimal cluster:

Physical state — Optimal cluster:

A 0 1 2 3 4 5
B 0 1 2 3 4 5
C 0 1 2 3 4 5
D 0 1 2 3 4 5
E 0 1 2 3 4 5

Mental state — Optimal cluster:

A 0 1 2 3 4 5
B 0 1 2 3 4 5
C 0 1 2 3 4 5
D 0 1 2 3 4 5
E 0 1 2 3 4 5

Quality of life — Optimal cluster:

A 0 1 2 3 4 5
B 0 1 2 3 4 5
C 0 1 2 3 4 5
D 0 1 2 3 4 5
E 0 1 2 3 4 5

Score:
Poor = 0   Very Good = 3
Fair = 1   Excellent = 4
Good = 2   Optimal = 5

FIGURE 16.2 (*continued*)

The scores for all of the components are added up to arrive at an aggregated figure of 0 (minimum) to 20.

The quality of life has a constant A which is predetermined for the community as a whole. The aggregate figure is added to A to arrive at the final result.

17
Use of a Functional Status Instrument in the Danish Health Study

N. Bentzen, K.M. Pedersen, and T. Christiansen

Introduction

To make sound decisions about the allocation of resources in the health care sector, it is important to obtain relevant knowledge about the incidence and prevalence of health problems in the population and the consequences of these problems in terms of use of resources and of personal discomfort. Furthermore, it is desirable that use of resources is related to course of treatment for a given illness, as opposed to being associated with each single contact to health providers or with bed-days. Moreover, it is desirable to be able to measure the effect of health care services on the health status of the target group.

In the Danish Health Study (DHS), the occurrence of health problems in the general population and subsequent actions taken from October 1982 to October 1983 have been registered in a longitudinal study using a health diary that was returned weekly. Courses of treatment are conceptualized as episodes of treatment, which are derived from episodes of illness. Data on health status have been obtained by using a series of questions related to different aspects of health. Data on health status were collected twice (October 1982 and November 1983) for adult panel members.

The DHS is based on a random sample of 1,321 Danish households with 3,419 members. An extensive background interview was conducted for these persons. Of these, 1,067 households, with 2,825 members, were recruited for a panel; members of the panel reported once a weak for a year through the use of health diaries. Diaries were used to register perceived health problems—their duration and consequences in terms of activity restrictions—self-care, professional care, and expenditures for professional care. At the end of the year (October 1983), the remaining panel members were given a closing interview by mail.

Compared to similar Danish survey studies, the DHS has some distinctly novel features. The sample unit in the random sample was the household, not the individual; background information was gathered for all individuals in a selected household; and the subsequent registration of health problems by means of a diary was equally detailed for all household members. This opens

236

up for analyses based on the household as the unit of analysis, along with analyses based on the individual as a unit. Moreover, the sample is not restricted to adults only but includes all age groups. In the study, traditional retrospective interviews have been combined with prospective data collection. Yet another feature is the elaborate registration of health status before and after the data collection with diaries.

Obectives of the Study

The aims of the current study are closely related and characterized by a general health economic approach (compare the frame of reference outlined below in Figure 17.1), yet may be summarized as addressing several distinct problem areas, as follow:

1. A description of the pattern of health problems in the Danish population and changes over time. The description is to include incidence and type of acute health problems, both new health problems and acute flare-ups of chronic conditions. In addition, prevalence and type of chronic health problems are to be described.

2. A description of illness and treatment episodes for selected health problems. This description is to include type of health problem, length of illness and treatment episodes, self-care, and professional care by type of provider.

3. A study of patient behavior in terms of self-care, professional care, or "alternative" care.

4. A study of time profiles of treatment episodes.

5. An investigation of the possibilities of applying a measure of health status to the Danish population.

6. A study of the relation between use of health services and health status as measured by the health status measure.

7. Formulation and estimation of models of demand and utilization based on the theory of demand for health. Here, health status should be included as an explanatory variable.

8. A study of costs of treatment of different health problems in terms of professional resources and the patient's own resources.

9. A study of the use of services related to the supply of health care services.

10. A study of the family as a basic provider of health care, based on models of household demand or utilization as opposed to models of individual behavior.

A Frame of Reference

The concepts of health status and illness and treatment episodes can be integrated in a frame of reference (Figure 17.1). Health status is regarded as either a dependent or an independent variable. It is influenced negatively by

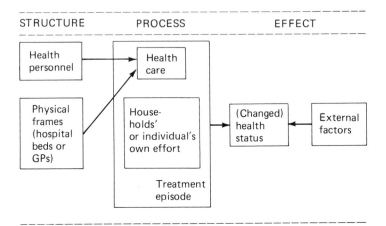

FIGURE 17.1. A frame of reference for the Danish Health Study. Reprinted with permission from (18).

illness episodes leading to a treatment episode. The treatment episode affects health status positively. Supply of health services in the region in which the household is located is assumed to influence duration and composition of the treatment episode.

Within such a frame of reference, it will be possible to analyze relations between occurrence of health problems and composition, duration, and time profile of treatment episodes along with a number of factors that are expected to influence the course of illness and treatment. Thus, socioeconomic conditions, working conditions, and health status of the individual, as well as health care services available, should be considered.

Alternatively, the relation between illness, treatment, and health status may be analyzed within a broad socioeconomic theory of demand for and use of health services. Demand for services may be viewed as derived from demand for health as a fundamental commodity. Within such a framework, factors influencing the production of and demand for health may be analyzed [compare the tradition of Becker–Grossman models (1, 2)].

In order to understand the course of illness and treatment episodes, it will be necessary to view the individual as part of a greater social entity: the family. It is obvious that the concept of children's demand for health care can only be understood in a family context. However, a family context may also be applied to adults. Thus, the family is assumed to function as the basic health care provider; within the family, a number of minor health problems are solved, and it is here that a decision about seeking professional health care takes place.

Important Topics of the Study

The important topics of this study are measurement of health status and use of concepts of illness and treatment episodes. For various reasons, there is a specific interest in a study of each of those two topics, but—as it can be inferred from the frame of reference—the analysis of some questions, that is, demand for treatment episodes, requires that both are included along with relevant background information.

Health Status Measurement

REASONS FOR INCLUDING HEALTH STATUS

As seen in some works on health economics, there is theoretical, and empirical, interest in the subject of health status measurement. Alan Williams (3) tried to grapple with the relationship among welfare economics, and health status measurement. Manning, Newhouse, and Ware (4) show that much is gained by using health status scales or indices in empirical demand studies instead of the customary question about being "excellent".... "poor." Sintonen (5) has attempted to include a health status measure in a resource allocation formula in order to capture the consumption benefit aspect of medical care.

Apart from the intrinsic relevance for health economics, there is a separate interest in health status measures that capture more than the traditional mortality and morbidity measures. In particular, there is a great and pressing need to include health status measures in population surveys of utilization of health services and other health-related matters.

There are two main arguments for the inclusion of health status measurement in the DHS. First, based on the utilization and cost data collected, it is one of the study's purposes to estimate demand models in the Grossman tradition (2) and according to more traditional "utilization models." In both cases, a measure of health status is needed. When the project was planned, it was decided that simple statements such as "my health is excellent,...." were insufficient and in no way mirrored the rather broad health concept implied in Grossman's work.* This belief has been confirmed retrospectively by Manning et al. (4), who investigated what is to be gained by using more refined measures of health† and what the consequences are of using current health to explain past utilization behavior.‡ Second, the project group wanted to test and/or construct a health status index in a general population survey, in part to ascertain whether it is possible, in part to gain experience in health status measurement.

---

*See Pedersen et al. (6) for an early attempt to use a more satisfactory (conceptually and technically) measure of health status in connection with demand for dental care.
†Namely, reliability, and hence less random measurement error, and comprehensiveness, possibly leading to reduced omitted variable bias.
‡Namely, inconsistency of the estimated regression coefficients.

CONSIDERATIONS BEFORE CHOOSING A SUITABLE INSTRUMENT

The group behind the Health Insurance Study (HIS) has published a number of points concerning choice of instrument for measuring health status (7), and since they closely resemble the prior reasoning of the project group, they will be the basis of discussion here:

1. Before selecting measures, the reason for studing health status must be identified.

2. When an instrument is selected, the concept of health must be clear. Thus, the health concept to the used must be identified unambiguously. It is believed that health is a multidimensional concept—and despite the much criticized WHO definition of health, the concept used must and should be close to that: a state of complete physical, mental, and social well-being and not merely the absence of disease and infirmity (8). The important aspects here are the three dimensions: physical, mental and social. Furthermore, it was believed that health should be measured in behavioral terms. The idea may be clarified by the following two excerpts from writings on the subject:

...health or function status should be defined and measured in terms of behavioural functioning. There are two reasons for this. One relates to the problems of reliability and validity associated with non-behavioural measures, such as perceived health and self-diagnosis. The other is that it is in terms of behavioural functioning rather than perceived health or diagnosis (self or medical) that the concept of health is most relevant to social system functioning (9).

The developers of the Sickness Impact Profile (SIP) note that

Behaviour is the single most important indicator of sickness in that it reflects the total impact of illness, including its clinical and subjective dimensions. Further, the functioning of an individual in terms of activities is the ultimate sought product of health care (10).

In the DHS, it was assumed that (i) health is multidimensional and (ii) behavioral measures in terms of functioning should be included. Also, (iii) the third issue is related to suitability of available instruments. Seven points must be observed here.

1. Practicality in terms of administration, respondent burden, and analysis. Keywords are "self-administration versus interviewing," "scaling methods involving judges verus nonjudge methods," and "ease of use in practical work."

2. Reliability in terms of the study design and group or individual comparison, that is, reliability of indices constructed.

3. Validity in terms of providing information about the relevant health dimension.

4. Sensitivity, that is, ability to measure changes taking place over time. Following Sintonen's list (5), three other points can be added.

5. The measure should be disease and program independent, that is, it should allow comparisons across disease categories and agency lines.

6. The measure should be understandable in the sense that the data to be

used to compute the measure and the process of computing should be readily understandable not only by those who will supposedly be using the measure, for instance, planners, but also by those who will supposedly be influenced by the measures, that is, decision makers and the general public.

7. It should be possible to relate the measures to variables over which health policy has some control.

THE ACTUAL CHOICE OF INSTRUMENT

During the planning phase, it was realized that it was not possible for a small group of researchers to develop their own health status measure, particularly since a number of other novel features of the study were considered to be more important. It was found that the field of health status measurement had progressed far enough that it was preferable to use an already existing instrument.

If the above list of rather formidable requirements is applied strictly to the available measures, none would pass on all counts. However, an inspection pointed towards two measures that had been thoroughly tested for validity and reliability—and they also appeared to be rather sensitive to changes in health status over time. The two instruments were the SIP (10) and the HIS (11, 12). They differ in one important respect—that of practicability. The SIP measure can be used in self-administered and interviewing form, but, in contrast to the HIS measure, the scaling method presupposes the use of judges, which is both time consuming and expensive, or the use of weights obtained in other surveys. Both measures are multidimensional and both are valid and reliable. Based primarily on practical grounds, the HIS measure was selected for testing in the pilot study—and subsequently adopted in the DHS.*

Another consideration of relevance when adopting a particular instrument is the danger of adopting "culture-specific" instruments. This is clearly an issue in the present context, since both SIP and HIS were developed in the United States. This issue was evaluated specifically for the HIS instrument. The method used may be described as an inspection of the questions entering the various scales with respect to face validity in a Danish context. It must be emphasized that this process by its very nature is subjective and must be based on relatively good knowledge of both the national and the foreign "culture." Based on this approach, it was decided (on hindsight probably unwise) to drop the mental health section in the pilot survey, and a few questions were deleted from the social health section. With respect to the mental health battery, two reasons for rejection may be noted: it was felt that the questions were "too American," for instance, a question like "How happy, satisfied, or pleased have you been with your presonal life?"

The reason for rejection was also related to the question of proper translation, not in the literal sense but rather in the sense of capturing the

---

*See reference 13 for results from the pilot study.

meaning and intention of the question. As an example, the reader might contemplate how to translate the above question in such a way that he or she would be willing and able to ask the question without feeling somewhat silly — or consider how to capture the meaning of the following: "Have you felt downhearted and blue...?" *Blue* is a state of mind that almost escapes direct translation. Translation, literal as well as "meaningful," is undoubtedly a greater problem than many think. For instance, Donald Patrick in a personal conversation has recounted how difficult it was to translate the American English in the SIP into British English; one crucial test was an attempt to retranslate the result. In some cases, it was rather difficult to recognize the retranslated American–English question.

Two questions about church activities were dropped from the social dimension because churchgoing and church activities are of a different nature in the United States than in Denmark. No attempt was made to substitute new questions.

An attempt to include the mental health battery probably should have been made because it was found that the rest of the HIS instrument appears to be surprisingly "culture insensitive," that is, it is of rather general applicability. In the DHS, a mental health dimension with 22 items from a "psychic vulnerability test" ("psykisk sårbarhedstest") was included. It has been thoroughly tested in Denmark (14, 15) with respect to reliability, validity, and scalability.* In view of the fact that the discussion of the HIS mental health index stressed that mental health involves both negative aspects (anxiety and depression) and positive aspects (optimism, self control), views with which the project group agreed, it was decided, in view of the good experience with other parts of the HIS instrument in the pilot study, that the HIS questions pertaining to, among other things, what the RAND researchers have termed positive well-being should be included. Hence, 10 items were added to the 22 items, 5 of which capture clearly positive aspects. The 32 questions have yes/no answer categories in contrast to the graduated six-point scale used by the HIS researchers.

It is hypothesized that health status is best captured through the behavioral–functional approach. There is no doubt that health perceptions are relevant for a number of health actions. For instance, it seems likely that resistance, susceptibility, and attitude toward seeing a doctor are important determinants of "self-care behavior," that is, in explaining why some persons, with the same symptom severity, choose to care for themselves, while others enter the health care system. Also, one might expect that health perceptions are determined, at least in part, by the behavioral-based health status measures.

To test these ideas, it was decided to include the HIS section on health perceptions.

---

*The original source of the test is identical to the "twenty-two item battery" developed during World War II by the now famous Stoufer group [see Measurement and Prediction (16)].

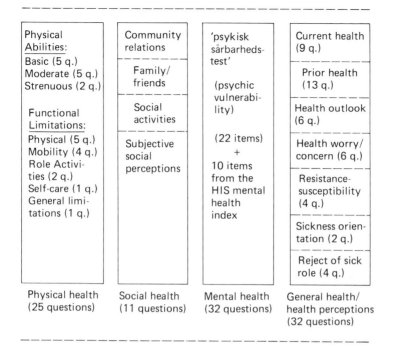

Physical Abilities: Basic (5 q.) Moderate (5 q.) Strenuous (2 q.) Functional Limitations: Physical (5 q.) Mobility (4 q.) Role Activities (2 q.) Self-care (1 q.) General limitations (1 q.)	Community relations Family/ friends Social activities Subjective social perceptions	'psykisk sårbarhedstest' (psychic vulnerability) (22 items) + 10 items from the HIS mental health index	Current health (9 q.) Prior health (13 q.) Health outlook (6 q.) Health worry/ concern (6 q.) Resistance-susceptibility (4 q.) Sickness orientation (2 q.) Reject of sick role (4 q.)
Physical health (25 questions)	Social health (11 questions)	Mental health (32 questions)	General health/ health perceptions (32 questions)

FIGURE 17.2. The four dimensions of health, the constituent hypothesized components, and the number of items involved. Reprinted with permission from (18).

In the DHS, health has been conceptualized as consisting of four dimensions, each one made up of a number of components. Figure 17.2 is an attempt to depict the various dimensions and components. With respect to the first three dimensions, "functioning" is measured. "General health," or health perception, makes up the fourth dimension.

Health is a latent variable or trait.* Therefore, health must be measured; thus, a number of questions or items must be used to elicit information on the latent variable (variables). The questionnaire containing questions about health status is shown in the Appendix. The total number of questions add up to no less than 100, which shows that in terms of interviewing time or self-administration, considerable time is involved, in particular when the health status battery is embedded in a general background interview, as was the case in the DHS.

In practice, the sequence of questions is determined by the four dimensions. Within dimensions, however, the questions related to the various components may be presented ramdomly to avoid any sequence effect. Thus, the

---

*This feature is further discussed in Bentzen et al. (17) where Rasch's measurement model is used for statistical analysis.

component making up the various dimensions are in reality hypotheses to be confirmed in the subsequent scaling analyses.

No overall health status index, that is, an index made up of all the dimensions or components, has been envisaged, as indicated in Figure 17.2.

The health status of children was not measured during the initial interview. A set of questions developed in the HIS study (7) appeared to be very difficult to administer within reasonable time limits. A small battery was included in the November 1983 closing interview on children's health status.

Frequency distribution of the health status measurement prior to the investigation period is shown in the Appendix, which also includes the postal questionnaire on children's health status (pp. 246–262).

Frequency distribution of the health status measurement after the data collection period (one-year diary period) is not included in this chapter but is published in "The Danish Health Study, design, questionnaire, health diary, validation and frequency distribution" (18).

Concluding Remarks

The unique characteristics of the design of this study is a combination of cross-sectional and longitudinal data from a panel that reported weekly throughout a whole year. Although cross-sectional data were obtained during personal interviews and by a postal questionnaire, longitudinal data were obtained through the use of a health diary. Methodological studies has shown that, in general, the diary has advantages over retrospective interviews with respect to levels of reporting, recording errors, and validation of health reports. Furthermore, such data have analytical advantages in that they allow health problems and their development over time and the consequence of actions taken to be studied.

This study shows that it is possible to recruit and maintain a panel for a period of one year without a substantial number of drop outs. Drop out especially took place in the beginning of the reporting period; it was related to the efforts made during the data collection phase to motivate the respondents to keep their diaries and return them on time. It has been demonstrated that no significant change in the level of reporting took place during the rest of the year. This indicates that the respondents did not become tired of or careless with their health diaries.

In general the validity of data from the diaries seems acceptable. Validation of the health status measured will be published in a separate report.

References

1. Becker GS. A theory of the allocation of time. *Econ J* 75:495–517, 1965.
2. Grossman M. The demand for health: A theoretical and empirical investigation. Ocassional paper, NBER; New York; 1972:119.

3. Williams A. Welfare economics and health status measurement. *Publ Hlth Rep* 82:271–282, 1987.

4. Manning WG, Newhouse JP, Ware JE. The status of health in demand estimation: or beyond excellent, good, fair, poor, In Fuchs VR (ed); Economic Aspects of Health, pp. 143–184, Chicago, 1982.

5. Sintonen H. *An Approach to Economic Evaluation of Actions for Health.* Helsinki, Finland: 1981. Ministry of Social Affairs and Health, Research Department.

6. Pedersen KM, Petersen PE. The demand for dental care among industrial workers: Construction and testing of a structural model. In: Working papers No. 6/1980, Institute of Social Science; Odense University, 1980.

7. Ware JE, Book RH, Davies AR, Lohr KN. Choosing Measures of health status for individuals in general populations. *Am J Publ Hlth* 71(6):620–625, 1981.

8. The World Health Organization Constitution. Geneva; 1948.

9. Roghman KJ, Haggerty RJ. Family stress and the use of health services. *Int J Epidemiol* 1(3):279–286, 1972.

10. Gilson BS, Bergner M, Bobitt RA, Carter WB. The Sickness Impact Profile: Final development and testing. Discussion Paper No 14, Center for Health Services Research, November 1979. (See Med. Care 19(8):787–805, 1981 for a reproduction of the main part of the discussion paper).

11. Brook RH, Ware JE Jr, Davies-Avery A, et al. Overview of adult health status measures fielded in Rand's Health Insurance Study. *Med Care* 17(7):1–129, 1979.

12. Brook RH, Ware JE, et al. (in various order in various volumes). Conceptualization and measurement of health for adults. In: The Health Insurance Study; Vols. I–VII, 1979–1980; Rand Corporation; Santa Monica, Calif.

13. Bentzen N, Christiansen T, Pedersen KM. Duration of character of illness and treatment episodes in the Danish population related to health status, socioeconomic conditions and regional supply of health services: A pilot study [in Danish]. Odense, Denmark; August 1981 (Unpublished data).

14. Andersen EB, Sørensen SL. Measurement of psychological vulnerability. An analysis of certain characteristics of the vulnerability test [in Danish]. Research report No. 58: Dept. of Statistics; 1979; University of Copenhagen.

15. Kühl P-H, Martini S. Psychologically vulnerable persons, their social- and living conditions [in Danish]. Publ. No. 102: The National Institute of Social Research, Copenhagen; 1981.

16. Stouffer SA, Guttman L, Suchman EA, Lazarsfeld PF, Star SA, Clausen JA. *Measurement and prediction.* Princeton, NJ: Princeton University Press; 1950 (Republished Wiley and Sons; 1966).

17. Bentzen N, Christiansen T, Pedersen KM. Measurement of health status in a general population survey: Choice of instrument. Issues in scaling. Occasional Papers, Dept. of Public Finance and Policy: Odense University; 1985:19.

18. Bentzen N, Christiansen T, Pedersen KM. The Danish Health Study. Design, questionnaire, health diary, validation and frequency distributions. Occasional paper, Odense University; 1988:3.

Appendix*

Translated questionnaires with univariate frequency distributions.
  Questionnaires used in the initial interview about health status:

1. Functional limitations
2. Physical abilities
3. Social activities
4. Health perceptions
5. General well-being (mental health)

  Questionnaires used in the closing postal interview:

1. Child health status
2. Health status (similar to the above—and omitted here) (18)

Household reference number: ——
Are you (indicate by x)
☐ Housewife
☐ Husband

FUNCTIONAL LIMITATIONS

In the following, a number of questions will be asked about limitations of your activities, due to your health. Please indicate by X at each question.

1. Are you unable to drive a car because of your health?

%

| 3.4 | Yes, unable to drive a car because of health |

How long have you been unable to drive a car because of your health?

%

1.7	Less than 1 month
3.4	1–3 months
94.8	More than 3 months

| 96.6 | No |

$n = 2,241$ $n = 58$

2. When you travel around your community, does someone have to assist you because of your health?

%

| 1.7 | Yes |

How long have you needed someone to assist you in travelling around your community?

*Adapted from Health Insurance Study (HIS).

%

98.3	No

%	
5.4	Less than 1 month
2.7	1–3 months
91.9	More than 3 months

$n = 2,223$ $n = 37$

3. Do you have to stay indoors most or all of the day because of your helath?

%

2.0	Yes

How long have you had to stay indoors most or all of the day because of your health?

%

98.0	No

%	
15.9	Less than 1 month
4.5	1–3 months
79.5	More than 3 months

$n = 2,222$ $n = 44$

4. Are you in bed or a chair for most or all of the day because of your health?

%

1.4	Yes

How long have you been in bed or a chair most or all of the day because of your health?

%

98.6	No

%	
16.7	Less than 1 month
6.7	1–3 months
76.5	More than 3 months

$n = 2,219$ $n = 30$

5. Does your health limit the kind of vigorous activities you can do, such as running, lifting heavy objects, or participating in strenuous sports?

%

20.1	Yes

How long has your health limited the kind of vigorous activities you can do?

%

79.9	No

%	
1.6	Less than 1 month
4.4	1–3 months
94.0	More than 3 months

$n = 2,221$ $n = 435$

6. Do you have any trouble either walking 1 km or walking upstairs to the 3rd floor?

%

8.4	Yes

How long have you had trouble either walking 1 km or walking upstairs to the 3rd floor?

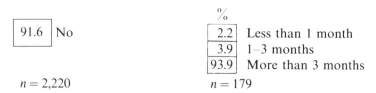

%	
91.6 No	2.2 Less than 1 month
	3.9 1–3 months
	93.9 More than 3 months
n = 2,220	n = 179

7. Do you have trouble bending or lifting because of your health?

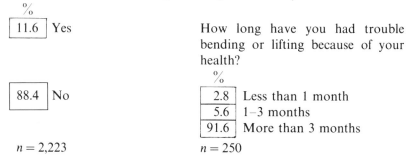

%

11.6 Yes

How long have you had trouble bending or lifting because of your health?

%

88.4 No

2.8	Less than 1 month
5.6	1–3 months
91.6	More than 3 months

n = 2,223   n = 250

8. Do you have any trouble either walking 100 m or climbing one flight of stairs because of your health?

%

2.8 Yes

How long have you had trouble either walking 100 m or climbing one flight of stairs because of your health?

%

97.2 No

3.5	Less than 1 month
3.5	1–3 months
93.0	More than 3 months

n = 2,221   n = 57

9. Are you unable to walk unless you are assisted by another person or by cane, crutches, artificial limbs, or braces?

%

2.2 Yes

How long have you been unable to walk without assistance?

%

97.8 No

—	Less than 1 month
4.4	1–3 months
95.6	More than 3 months

n = 2,223   n = 45

10. Are you unable to do certain kinds or amounts of work, housework, or school work because of your health?

%

6.2 Yes

How long have you been unable to do certain kinds or amounts of work, housework, or schoolwork because of your health?

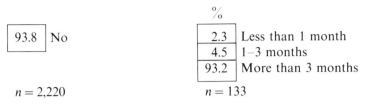

%

| 93.8 | No |

n = 2,220

2.3	Less than 1 month
4.5	1–3 months
93.2	More than 3 months

n = 133

11. Does your health keep you from working at a job, doing work around the house, or going to school?

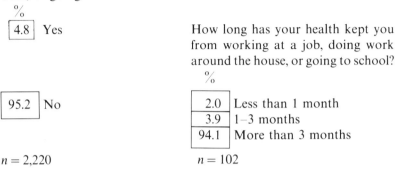

%

| 4.8 | Yes |

How long has your health kept you from working at a job, doing work around the house, or going to school?

%

| 95.2 | No |

2.0	Less than 1 month
3.9	1–3 months
94.1	More than 3 months

n = 2,220

n = 102

12. Do you need help with eating, dressing, bathing, or using the toilet because of your health?

%

| 0.6 | Yes |

How long have you needed help with eating dressing, bathing, or using the toilet because of your health?

%

| 99.4 | No |

—	Less than 1 month
15.4	1–3 months
84.6	More than 3 months

n = 2,223

n = 13

13. Does your health limit you in any way from doing anything you want to do?

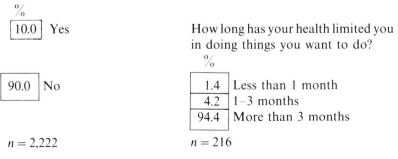

%

| 10.0 | Yes |

How long has your health limited you in doing things you want to do?

%

| 90.0 | No |

1.4	Less than 1 month
4.2	1–3 months
94.4	More than 3 months

n = 2,222

n = 216

PHYSICAL ACTIVITIES

The following questions are about physical limitations you might have

1. Can you participate in active sports such as soccer, handball, swimming, tennis or rowing a boat?

%
74.5 [ ] Yes–Q. 2
6.0 [ ] Yes, but cautiously } Why?
19.4 [ ] No _____
n = 2,248

%	Visual problems	Hearing problems	Bronchitis, asthma, breathing problems	Heart trouble	High blood pressure	Anemia	Back problem	Rheumatism in muscles	Arthritis	Other problems with muscles or joints	Stomach or intestinal illness	Varicose veins	Obesity	Diabetes	Bladder or kidney infections	Allergy, hay fever	Old age	Other	
Indicate by one X the most important cause	1.2	1.2	9.8	5.6	4.8	0.2	17.8	4.1	2.7	8.7	1.0	1.5	0.8	—	0.6	0.2	29.7	11.2	n = 518

2. Can you do hard activities at home like lifting or moving heavy furniture or spring cleaning?

%
80.5 [ ] Yes–Q. 3
7.3 [ ] Yes, but cautiously } Why?
12.2 [ ] No _____
n = 2,247

%	Visual problems	Hearing problems	Bronchitis, asthma, breathing problems	Heart trouble	High blood pressure	Anemia	Back problem	Rheumatism in muscles	Arthritis	Other problems with muscles or joints	Stomach or intestinal illness	Varicose veins	Obesity	Diabetes	Bladder or kidney infections	Allergy, hay fever	Old age	Other	
Indicate by one X the most important cause	0.3	0.3	6.0	5.8	5.0	0.3	37.7	4.2	2.6	7.9	1.0	0.5	0.3	—	0.5	—	22.3	5.5	n = 382

If you have answered yes unconditionally in question 1 and question 2 the rest of this page can be skipped.

3. Can you do moderate work at home like moving a chair or pushing a vacuum cleaner?

%
85.3 [ ] Yes–Q. 4
8.8 [ ] Yes, but cautiously } Why?
6.0 [ ] No _____
n = 604

%	Visual problems	Hearing problems	Bronchitis, asthma, breathing problems	Heart trouble	High blood pressure	Anemia	Back problem	Rheumatism in muscles	Arthritis	Other problems with muscles or joints	Stomach or intestinal illness	Varicose veins	Obesity	Diabetes	Bladder or kidney infections	Allergy, hay fever	Old age	Other	
Indicate by one X the most important cause	—	—	6.3	9.5	3.2	1.6	36.5	3.2	4.8	4.8	1.6	—	—	—	—	—	22.2	6.3	n = 63

4. Can you do light work around the house like dusting or washing dishes?

%
- 95.4 — Yes–Q. 5
- 2.5 — Yes, but cautiously } Why?
- 2.2 — No
- n = 604

□ 6.3 □ — □ 12.5 □ 18.8 □ — □ 6.3

Indicate by one X the most important cause

□ 12.5 □ — □ 6.3 □ — □ — □ — □ — □ 37.5 □ —

n = 16

5. If you wanted to could you run a short distance?

%
- 49.1 — Yes–Q. 6
- 10.9 — Yes, but cautiously } Why?
- 40.0 — No
- n = 605

□ — □ 14.9 □ 10.4 □ 5.2 □ 0.4

Indicate by one X the most important cause

□ 9.0 □ 3.4 □ 4.1 □ 8.2 □ 1.5 □ 1.1 □ 1.5 □ 0.4 □ 28.4 □ 11.2

n = 268

6. Can you walk uphill or up stairs?

%
- 77.1 — Yes–Q. 7
- 15.4 — Yes, but cautiously } Why?
- 7.5 — No
- n = 603

□ — □ 0.9 □ 12.2 □ 5.2 □ 1.9

Indicate by one X the most important cause

□ 7.0 □ 5.2 □ 3.5 □ 9.6 □ 1.7 □ 0.9 □ 1.7 □ 0.9 □ 19.1 □ 8.7

n = 115

7. Can you walk a distance of at least 1/2 km?

%
- 80.6 — Yes–Q. 8
- 11.4 — Yes, but cautiously } Why?
- 7.9 — No
- n = 604

□ — □ — □ 7.2 □ 7.2 □ 1.0

Indicate by one X the most important cause

□ 10.3 □ 2.1 □ 6.2 □ 13.4 □ 1.0 □ 1.0 □ 2.1 □ — □ 24.7 □ 9.3

n = 97

8. Can you walk around inside the house?

%
- 97.7 — Yes–Q. 9
- 1.8 — Yes, but cautiously } Why?
- 0.5 — No
- n = 603

□ — □ — □ 11.1 □ 11.1 □ —

Indicate by one X the most important cause

□ 11.1 □ — □ — □ 11.1 □ — □ — □ — □ — □ 55.5 □ —

n = 9

(continued)

PHYSICAL ACTIVITIES

The following questions are about physical limitations you might have

	Visual problems	Hearing problems	Bronchitis, asthma, breathing problems	Heart trouble	High blood pressure	Anemia	Back problem	Rheumatism in muscles	Arthritis	Other problems with muscles or joints	Stomach or intestinal illness	Varicose veins	Obesity	Diabetes	Bladder or kidney infections	Allergy, hay fever	Old age	Other	
9. Can you walk to a table for meals? % 98.7 Yes–Q. 10; 0.8 Yes, but cautiously Why?; 0.5 No; n = 604	□ —	□ —	□ —	□ —	□ 25.0	□ —	□ 25.0	□ —	□ —	□ —	□ —	□ —	□ —	□ —	□ —	□ —	□ 50.0	□ —	n = 4
% Indicate by one X the most important cause																			
10. Can you dress yourself? % 98.2 Yes–Q. 11; 1.2 Yes, but cautiously Why?; 0.7 No; n = 604	□ —	□ —	□ —	□ —		□ —	□ 25.0	□ —	□ —	□ —	□ —	□ —	□ —	□ —	□ —	□ —	□ 75.0	□ —	n = 4
% Indicate by one X the most important cause																			
11. Can you eat without help? % 99.3 Yes–Q. 12; 0.3 Yes, but cautiously Why?; 0.3 No; n = 604	□ —	□ —	□ —	□ —	□ —	□ —	□ —	□ —	□ —	□ —	□ —	□ —	□ —	□ —	□ —	□ —	□ 100.0	□ —	n = 1
% Indicate by one X the most important cause																			
12. Can you use the toilet without help? % 99.0 Yes–Q. 13; 0.5 Yes, but cautiously Why?; 0.5 No; n = 604	□ —	□ —	□ —	□ —	□ —	□ —	□ —	□ —	□ —	□ —	□ —	□ —	□ —	□ —	□ —	□ —	□ 100.0	□ —	n = 3
% Indicate by one X the most important cause																			

SOCIAL ACTIVITIES

1. About how many families are you so well acquainted with that you visit each other in your homes?

   13.3 (Enter number of families) $n = 2,212$

2. About how many *close* friends do you have—people you feel at ease with and can talk with about what is on your mind? (You may include relatives.)

   9.4 (Enter number of close friends) $n = 2,132$

3. Over a year's time, about how often do you get together with friends and relatives, such as going out together or visiting in each other's homes?

   %

2.0	Every day
19.5	Several days a week
29.9	About once a week
24.2	2–3 times a month
13.9	About once a month
7.2	5–10 times a year
3.3	Less than 5 times a year

                                                                    $n = 2,247$

4. During the *past month*, about how often have you had friends over to your home? (Do *not* include relatives.)

   %

2.3	Every day
15.6	Several days a week
22.9	About once a week
33.0	2–3 times in the past month
15.1	Once in the past month
11.1	Not at all in the past month

                                                                    $n = 2,247$

5. About how often have you visited friends at their homes during the *past month*? (Do *not* count relatives.)

   %

0.4	Every day
10.6	Several days a week
20.9	About once a week
36.6	2–3 times in the past month
17.2	Once in the past month
14.3	Not at all in the past month

                                                                    $n = 2,245$

6. About how often were you on the telephone with close friends or relatives during the *past month?*

%

23.3	Every day
38.3	Several days a week
20.4	About once a week
11.7	2–3 times in the past month
3.1	Once in the past month
3.1	Not at all in the past month

$n = 2,243$

7. About how often did you write a letter to a friend or relative during the *past month?*

%

0.3	Every day
1.5	Several days a week
3.6	About once a week
9.2	2–3 times in the past month
14.7	Once in the past month
70.8	Not at all in the past month

$n = 2,245$

8. In general, how well are you getting along with other people these days— would you say better than usual, about the same, or not as well as usual?

%

3.0	Better than usual
95.8	About the same
1.2	Not as well as usual

$n = 2,241$

9. About how many voluntary groups, clubs, study circles or organizations do you belong to? (Enter number—if none, write O)

2.6	Groups or organizations

$n = 1,644$

10. How active are you in the affairs of these groups or clubs you belong to? (If you belong to a great many, just count those you feel closest to. If you don't belong to any, enter x in the box at the bottom).

%

17.3	Very active, attend most meetings
28.4	Fairly active, attend fairly often
28.0	Not active, belong, but hardly ever go
26.2	Do not belong to any groups or clubs

$n = 2,229$

HEALTH PERCEPTIONS

The following statements are about your health. Please indicate to what extent you agree or disagree with each statement. Please enter X in the box you think is most true for you.

(Notice that there are no right or wrong answers. And don't think over each statement too long, but indicate your spontaneous answer by X).

	Agree entirely %	Agree %	Don't know %	Disagree %	Disagree entirely %	n
1. According to the doctors I have seen, my health is now excellent.	51.8	29.9	7.8	7.2	3.4	2,245
2. I try to avoid letting illness interfere with my life.	51.5	35.2	6.3	3.5	3.6	2,239
3. I seem to get sick a little easier than other people.	4.8	3.3	10.7	32.0	49.2	2,241
4. I feel better now than I ever have before.	14.0	18.8	29.4	23.1	14.7	2,239
5. I well probably be sick a lot in the future.	1.8	5.4	27.0	28.4	37.5	2,236
6. I never worry about my health.	47.7	31.0	4.8	11.0	5.6	2,245

(continued)

Health Perceptions (*Continued*)

	Agree entirely %	Agree %	Don't know %	Disagree %	Disagree entirely %	n
7. Most people get sick a little easier than I do.	8.0	14.2	48.3	18.7	10.7	2,240
8. I don't like to go to the doctor.	18.5	19.0	7.5	33.2	21.8	2,239
9. I am somewhat ill.	5.5	10.2	6.9	35.6	41.7	2,238
10. In the future, I expect to have better health than other people I know.	5.6	8.7	54.3	18.7	12.7	2,239
11. I was so sick once I thought I might die.	10.9	7.3	4.9	22.5	54.4	2,236
12. I'am not as healthy now as I used to be.	6.3	12.4	6.4	34.5	40.3	2,237
13. I worry about my health more than others do.	3.4	6.0	23.6	29.6	37.4	2,237
14. When I'am sick, I try to just keep going as usual.	33.4	45.0	9.2	9.0	3.3	2,241

						N
15. My body seems to resist illness very well.	33.8	44.7	13.6	5.9	2.0	2,241
16. Getting sick once in a while is a part of my life.	6.1	16.5	10.1	34.5	32.9	2,232
17. I'm as healthy as anybody I know.	34.8	38.5	15.4	7.4	3.8	2,241
18. I think my health will be worse in the future than it is now.	2.3	7.7	37.7	26.6	25.7	2,239
19. I've never had an illness that lasted a long period of time.	40.9	26.7	2.6	19.9	13.9	2,234
20. Others seem more concerned about their health than I am about mine.	8.6	14.8	55.1	13.9	7.5	2,239
21. When I'am sick, I try to keep it to myself.	20.5	32.0	13.6	27.2	6.7	2,234
22. My health is excellent.	41.8	38.2	6.5	9.2	4.3	2,241
23. I expect to have a very healthy life.	26.9	30.7	31.9	7.7	2.8	2,249
24. My health is a concern in my life.	3.9	7.0	4.7	31.7	52.8	2,235

(continued)

Health Perceptions (*Continued*)

	Agree entirely %	Agree %	Don't know %	Disagree %	Disagree entirely %	n
25. I accept that sometimes I'm just going to be sick.	17.2	49.0	15.0	12.2	6.6	2,234
26. I have been feeling bad lately.	5.8	12.1	3.3	39.4	39.4	2,233
27. It doesn't bother me to go to a doctor.	33.0	34.6	5.0	17.0	10.5	2,239
28. I have never been seriously ill.	39.7	28.1	3.9	15.5	12.9	2,238
29. When there is something going around, I usually catch it.	4.2	7.2	15.1	40.0	33.7	2,237
30. Doctors say that I am now in poor health.	3.1	3.9	8.2	33.7	51.1	2,236
31. When I think I am getting sick, I fight it.	24.1	46.2	15.4	9.7	4.6	2,241
32. I feel about as good now as I ever had.	30.4	41.1	8.5	12.7	7.2	2,235

GENERAL WELL-BEING

The next questions are about your personal well-being. Do not think too much about each question, but give the answer you spontaneously think is most correct.

	Yes %	No %		
1.	11.5	88.5	Do you easily get "trembling hands?"	$n = 2{,}247$
2.	4.0	96.0	Do you often suffer from lack of appetite?	$n = 2{,}246$
3.	15.4	84.6	Do you often suffer from spells of bad headache?	$n = 2{,}242$
4.	14.3	85.7	Do you often have sleeping problems?	$n = 2{,}241$
5.	4.8	95.2	Do you often have spells of anxiety?	$n = 2{,}243$
6.	21.4	78.6	Are you often very tired?	$n = 2{,}238$
7.	16.8	83.2	Do you often take pills, for instance sleeping pills?	$n = 2{,}239$
8.	28.7	71.3	Do you often have pains, for instance chest or stomach pains?	$n = 2{,}235$
9.	4.9	95.1	Are you often nervous?	$n = 2{,}245$
10.	6.3	93.7	Do you often have spells of dizzines?	$n = 2{,}247$
11.	10.8	89.2	Do you think that noise bothers you more than it bothers other people?	$n = 2{,}243$
12.	2.0	98.0	Are you almost always in low spirits?	$n = 2{,}243$
13.	14.1	85.9	Do you have problems concentrating on your work when somebody is looking at you?	$n = 2{,}242$

(continued)

General well-being (*Continued*)

	Yes %	No %		
14.	7.5	92.5	Do your heart often beat very fast without any specific reason?	$n = 2,241$
15.	7.1	92.9	Do you often feel poorly?	$n = 2,240$
16.	4.4	95.6	Do you have problems making friends?	$n = 2,237$
17.	54.0	46.0	Do you find it difficult to accept that others control you/make decisions for you?	$n = 2,237$
18.	19.1	80.9	Do you prefer to keep to yourself?	$n = 2,216$
19.	10.1	89.9	Do small things bother you/get to you?	$n = 2,239$
20.	11.8	88.2	Do you constantly have thoughts that torment and make you uneasy?	$n = 2,237$
21.	21.9	78.1	Are you very shy and sensitive?	$n = 2,230$
22.	4.9	95.1	Do you often feel misunderstood by others?	$n = 2,239$
23.	81.1	18.9	Are you usually happy and satisfied with your life?	$n = 2,235$
24.	12.5	87.5	Do you often feel that you have nothing to look forward to?	$n = 2,238$
25.	90.9	9.1	Do you often feel that your life is full of things that interest you?	$n = 2,234$
26.	92.4	7.6	Do you often feel satisfied with carrying out your daily work?	$n = 2,228$
27.	7.7	92.3	Do you often feel downhearted and blue?	$n = 2,241$
28.	89.1	10.9	Do you usually feel cheerful, lighthearted about the future?	$n = 2,220$

General well-being (*Continued*)

Yes %	No %		
8.7	91.3	29. Do you often feel that things do not work out the way you want them?	$n = 2,235$
78.6	21.4	30. When you get up in the morning, do you often feel that you are looking forward to an interesting day?	$n = 2,206$
20.7	79.3	31. Are you often broody?	$n = 2,238$
17.3	82.7	32. Are you usually emotionally stable?	$n = 2,225$

Postal Questionnaire on Children's Health Status: To be answered for all children living at home

	Oldest child	Child no. 2	Child no. 3	Child no. 4
Overall, how do you evaluate your child's/children's health?	%	%	%	%
Good	85.7	85.6	88.7	100.0
Fairly good	9.5	8.9	8.6	—
Satisfactory	4.0	5.2	3.2	—
Relatively poor	0.9	0.4	—	—
Poor	—	—	—	—
	$n = 454$	$n = 271$	$n = 62$	$n = 5$
How, do you evaluate your child's/children's health compared to other children of the same age?	%	%	%	%
Better	22.0	19.2	16.1	—
About the same	75.6	77.5	80.6	100.0
Worse	2.4	3.3	3.2	—
	$n = 454$	$n = 271$	$n = 62$	$n = 5$
Have any of your children a lasting or chronic illness that demands long-term treatment or control (for example, diabetes?)	%	%	%	%
No	94.1	94.8	96.0	100.0
Yes	5.9	5.2	3.2	—
Enter which ———	$n = 454$	$n = 271$	$n = 62$	$n = 5$
Are any of your children disabled? (For example, hearing disability or physical handicap)	%	%	%	%
No	96.0	97.0	95.2	100.0
Yes	4.0	3.0	4.8	—
Enter which ———	$n = 454$	$n = 271$	$n = 62$	$n = 5$

Index